REQUIRED READING
FOR
THE WHOLE CANCER THING

An Insider's Tale

Plus

101 "Must Have" Survival Tips

Written by

Anne Kruse, M.S.

ISBN-13: 978-1508669234

ISBN-10: 1508669236

Published by Sisterhaus Publishing

Edited by Neetnik Editing

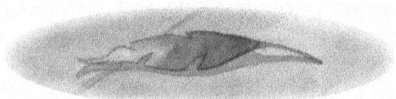

For More Information About The Author and Other Projects

Please Go To:

http://www.annekrusethewriter.com

Contact by e-mail: annekrusewriter@gmail.com

DEDICATION

To Michelle for listening to that small voice.

To Deborah for helping me believe in mine.

To my mom who proved there is life after cancer.

To Barb for showing me what living life means.

TABLE OF CONTENTS

INTRODUCTION

"There is no greater agony than bearing
an untold story inside you."

-Maya Angelou

The type of book I wanted to read prior to and/or while going through the cancer experience would have been a direct, informative, reality-based book with plenty of humor and a little snarky-ness peppered in to lighten the mood. I would have appreciated real information that included bad and good news and everything in-between. I would have loved to receive some warnings about certain things. I would have welcomed a real, "Truth Teller" into my corner. That's the kind of book I would have wanted; so that's the type of book I wrote. You can count on it.

No one gave me a roadmap for my voyage through cancer diagnosis, surgery, chemotherapy, radiation, recovery and rejuvenation. I believe in the power of storytelling. I'm telling my story to serve as a navigation tool for anyone who might be seeking direction. I will discuss "the stuff" you need to know that others may not tell you. Plenty of people believe that asking questions of someone going through the cancer experience is impolite, or at minimum uncomfortable. You know as well as I do, most people really do want to ask questions, and definitely are interested in the answers. I'm not saying people are nosey; or maybe they are. I appreciate a genuine curiosity about the human experience. I welcome all "appreciators" to read on.

It's true that everyone's journey is different; and this story is about mine. However, there are universal truths shared by everyone going through the cancer expedition. I decided to write this book not only because I wanted to, but because I had to. The physical and emotional experience I endured left me with a need to process its impact; and writing this book allowed me to do just that. When I received the cancer diagnosis, I thought it was the final blow that would stop my writing career once and for all. It felt like it was an ultimate tap on the shoulder and whisper in my ear saying, "It's not going to happen for you. The door is shutting." Writing each word of this book helped prop the door open.

Notes were tediously kept from the beginning and throughout my adventure. I knew I would be writing a book someday. How does anyone find their way to that *someday*? I just kept writing; and proved to myself I can write my way into and out of anything. This confidence was earned; and I relish the moments when I get to utilize the best parts of who I am to convey something so meaningful.

I have always found the question, "How long did it take you to write your book?" to be provocative. The answer to that question brings another question: isn't it true that writing any book takes your entire life to write? It's taken all my life-experience to get into *this* current life-space to write *this* story. Putting ink on the page commenced on December 29, 2013, the two-year anniversary of receiving a cancer diagnosis. Happy holidays to me. I finished writing this book January 25th, 2015, the three-year anniversary of my surgery to remove a large cancerous mass from my cervix, thirty-eight lymph nodes (one cancerous), my uterus and ovaries. This date served as both a deadline and a celebration of on-going recovery.

It is interesting how many people say, "I should write a book." It is also no surprise the majority never do. That is sad; and I understand it better than most. I knew I wanted to write my book but was feeling apprehensive. I attributed it to not being ready to dive in and write. The probability of impending doom was still too close to home. Was I going to be alive? I didn't want to start the book and not be able to finish. Dying would be depressing enough. I definitely didn't want to be remembered for not finishing a book. These were very real thoughts and feelings weighing heavily upon my motivation and progress. I will always remember the story about Jonathan Larson who wrote the wildly successful play *Rent*. He died unexpectedly from an aneurysm at one of the rehearsals before the debut and never got to see his dream come true. That story has always hit me hard in the stomach; and will always be one of the saddest stories I've ever heard.

I chose one of my favorite Maya Angelou quotes to open this Introduction: "There is no greater agony than bearing an untold story inside you." Maya Angelou was alive and still actively telling her stories when I began writing this book. She passed away May 28th, 2014, which was the impetus for the final push to finish. Writing this book definitely alleviated the agony of bearing the untold story inside of me. Sharing it with all of you is a profound experience - one that I'm looking forward to with great excitement.

My mother once told me the reason certain melodies make us cry is because they somehow speak to the divine part of our soul that has not been fully realized, been silenced or is patiently waiting a turn. Funny, I can simply think about that in utter silence with no peep of a melody and I get misty. I believe the agony Maya Angelou mentions finds its source in that same part of our being. Writing this book is part of my plan to let my soul out to sing for a while through storytelling: the greatest way to connect ourselves to humanity.

Pursuing a writing career will end up being my most brilliant move or the stupidest thing I've ever done. It made perfect sense to take my master's degree in psychology plus seventeen years of counseling experience, and combine it with UCLA's best-in-the-nation screenwriting graduate program to ultimately write meaty, relevant, intelligent and comedic roles for women. My plan was to populate feature films, television screens, or teeny-tiny screen mobile devices with *real* women characters. The pursuit of a writing career never makes perfect sense. While relentlessly toggling between my "brilliant move" and "the stupidest thing ever" feelings, I wrote movie and TV scripts, a children's book, newspaper and website articles, business bios, and then I got cancer. It looked like the meatiest, most relevant role to be written would be my own.

The scripts I write are intended to be performed and thus contain dialogue to be spoken. Dialogue doesn't always adhere to a keen sense of the Queen's English, and some of my stories may do the same to preserve a certain storytelling flare.

The Library of Congress separates literary works from screenplays when it comes to copyrighting material. Movies, television, and plays are meant to be performed for other humans to see. A book is filled with black ink on a page that must be read and processed and understood; and the reader must conjure up visuals in their own mind to fully experience it. My genetically-German knack for efficiency tells me watching a performance saves a lot of time and effort. However, I've realized a script that doesn't get produced and acted out by humans is very similar to a book, with one BIG exception. A book has a *full life* when it is read. Sadly, unproduced scripts die on the vine oozing potential, and fall short of a fully-expressed life. Each unproduced script must bear the agony of an untold story. It's sad, isn't it?

Will this book ever become a movie, piece of performance art or a musical? Not likely. Once I finished writing this book, I discovered I really needed to rewrite this Introduction. The writing experience changed my beliefs about books, amongst other things. My hope is that it will satisfy those who want an emotional, full-spectrum experience in which you find yourself crying, laughing, horrified, satisfied and everything in-between. Humbly speaking, that's what it did for me.

Required Reading for The Whole Cancer Thing. An Insider's Tale Plus 101 "Must Have" Survival Tips, is the title of this book and it warrants some elaboration.

When I refer to a very complex and involved struggle I've had in life, I hyper-condense it in conversations by saying, "The whole _____ thing." Some examples from my life include: the whole meth-addicted boss thing; the whole governor cancelling my program thing; the whole trying to be a writer thing. It serves as a way of communicating a huge life event in one sentence. How's that for efficient? It conveniently shifts it into manageable terms; and definitely stifles the hijacking of all the gray matter in my head.

My plan is to share this book with patients, family members, friends, doctors, administrators, medical and nursing students, counseling grad students, medical assistant trainees, writers and film school attendees, and anyone who stands a chance to benefit from my story. Yes, I have a Master's degree in psychology and extensive experience counseling others, but this book shouldn't be considered *professional advice*. Instead welcome it as friendly, thought-provoking insights from someone who's been in the belly of the beast, was barfed up, and wrote all about it. Sometimes just hearing the story of one person who had a similar experience is enough comfort to get you through the struggle. Sure, there's a bit of "misery loves company" operating; but I would be remiss to discount the notion that the cancer experience includes a lot of "celebration loves company" as well.

A special place in my heart is reserved for counselors in training. Being a counselor for so many years allowed me certain insights about my journey. Each up-and-coming counselor must decide where he or she will apply their talents within the vast human population. It takes a special person to share their gift of intellect and compassion with those who are dealing with cancer. This book will provide you a glimpse into the realities a patient must endure, which many times results in a need for counseling. Talents are gifts to be used. Cancer grants you, the counselor, opportunities to use yours. By the way, Chapter 14 includes nine possible Master's thesis and/or Doctoral dissertation ideas. Feel free to imbibe from the stream of ideas.

Foremost in my mind was pricing this book so most every income bracket could afford it. Those who can't afford it could likely rely upon the kindness of strangers to kick in a little more than the cost of a latte to help someone struggling with cancer. Caffeine is important, but come on – priorities. Besides, I know most people have a few bucks in change lingering in that special coin-compartment of their car or under their seat mingling with a dried up french-fry and a faded gas receipt.

Please be warned that some subject matter may be inappropriate for children and even for me, but I had to write it anyway. I prejudged certain subject matter to be TMI (too much information). Therefore, metaphors and analogies were used to get my point across because it's easier; and frankly, metaphors and analogies are fun. At times you may find yourself wanting to skip ahead a line or two or simply shut your eyes. I know I did. Scientific information will be discussed but shouldn't scare you away. It's really, really interesting. To balance things out there will be humor along the way. It was, and still is my best defense against pretty much anything. Once you get past the downer of reading a book about cancer, you'll see there's a great story to behold. I can honestly tell you I have never been turned down by anyone when I ask, "You want to hear a really good story?" Seriously, people will stop working, silence a baby, and even put their phone down for a good story.

I wanted to do my Masters' thesis on the healing effects of humor. Unfortunately, my meth-addicted boss at the time was running the company into a black whole, and I had to get out as fast as I could. Instead of completing a thesis, I opted for the expeditious route and took comprehensive exams to complete my degree. My hope is that the humor in this book provides healing, which would reinforce the research hypothesis I sadly never got to investigate.

Reality tells us that with the good comes the bad, and then the good comes again. With the happy comes the sad only to return to happy again. The pendulum swings. This is a book that's not afraid to tell the story, but will always try to acknowledge the positive when it's real and warranted. Unfortunately, sometimes things just suck; and there's no candy-coating. I promise there will be no sugary syrup lingering at the bottom of any pages. Also, there will be no perpetuation of false hope, but guarded optimism will always prevail. Most importantly, celebrations, no matter how small, will be celebrated.

You will notice I kept exact names out of my book to protect some identities and privacy; but I did use the correct first names of those people who positively impacted my experience. You know who you are. Okay, there were two people whose first names were used and proved to be dreadful antagonists in my story. You'll have to read on to figure that out.

I wanted to write this book in a way that sounded conversational. One of the best compliments I receive is when someone reads something I wrote and says, "I can totally hear your voice." My goal would be for you to feel like we just sat down together over a beverage of your choice and I talked your ear off, but not in an annoying kind of way. Writing this book is a one-way communication; but the fact that you're reading, and in essence listening, makes the communication complete. My hope is to also do an audio version of this book. That way the reader will definitely hear my voice the way I intended it to be heard. In the meantime, humor me.

So sit back, grab a snack and that beverage, and let's talk.

Ch 1 - FROM NOTHING TO SOMETHING

Spending the summer of 2010 working for my brother at his design studio was a financial bright spot in the Great Recession. I was helping my brother, making a little money, and feeling like I was moving in a positive financial direction. I didn't realize it, but other things were taking a new direction too.

The majority of us know how minor health annoyances can be. We usually wait to see if they go away on their own. I have a dear friend who does the same thing with her car; and it actually works, sometimes. Even when the health annoyance lingers, we just chalk it up to it taking longer to heal. When I was young and experienced growing pains they always went away - which gave me a certain level of confidence about weird body changes. Goodness knows we have to deal with some really freakish things.

My symptoms started slowly as a minor annoyance. First, there was nothing more than a pinkish discharge. Then, I thought I had somehow developed the poor hygiene habits of a sixth grade boy when no one was looking. What else could explain the mysterious soiling in my under garments? One can't help but question one's sanity when things start happening for no apparent reason.

I thought my anatomy was losing its ability to be waterproof, and I was only in my forties. What hope did I have for my long-range goal of staying out of Super-Absorbent Depends until I was in my eighties? One's aging body is confusing to say the least. What do you chalk up to normal aging, and what is abnormal?

Most of us have been handed down physical oddities from our parents - some more icky than others. I felt like I was the genetic garbage can of the family. The only thing I inherited from my dearly departed father was a bag of his trouser socks. Low and behold it seemed I unwittingly inherited my father's skewing toward hemorrhoids, accompanied by a leaky anal sphincter from some other person in my family tree. It was discovered that the hemorrhoids resulted from the cancerous tumor pushing on neighboring organs; and the leaky anal sphincter wasn't really leaking. The tumor was producing fluid, hence the pink discharge, which inundated an area more accustom to being a dry environment. Get the picture? Sorry about that. It won't be the only thing you want to "un-see."

Minimizing things happening in our body is not a good practice. The lead up to my cancer diagnosis was an especially confusing time. I was in my forties, an age group racked with perplexity and many physiological occurrences that made me feel like I was a victim of body snatching.

I was building a reputation for being wrong. In fact, I had never been more wrong about so many things in my life. That started right at age forty when my vision started getting worse. While looking at a shampoo bottle in the shower one day I noticed the print was much smaller than it had been, and it was blurry. Up to that point in my life when I couldn't see something, I moved the object closer. Now, I was experiencing a one-hundred-eighty degree opposite. I had to move the shampoo bottle further away

2

to see it clearly. That really was counterintuitive and it always made me feel a little crazy. How could I be so wrong? I mean, completely wrong. If I was that wrong about the shampoo bottle, what else could I be wrong about? Apparently, doubt can move into the minds of the confident.

For almost a decade I found myself being forced to add things to a list of conditions I was going to have to "put up with" for the rest of my life. I had inherited dark circles under my eyes, freckles in a not-so-freckle-friendly culture, a horrible weakness in my lower spine, auto-immune thyroiditis, flatter than normal feet, and a propensity toward allowing joy to be sucked out of my life. With each item added to my list, I fought the urge to become completely disillusioned about aging.

After a history of normal Pap tests and negative Human Papilloma Virus (HPV) tests my symptoms continued, and worsened. I spent the better part of 2010-2011 chasing symptoms. Let me be clear about one thing: I do not like going to the doctor. It took everything I had to stay on course and try to get to the bottom of the mystery that was my body. Even my Nurse Practitioner called me an enigma.

I actually had never met Dr. F (keeping names anonymous) in my gynecologist's office, because I always saw Michelle, the Nurse Practitioner. This puts anyone at a disadvantage in a situation like mine. Dr. F came highly recommended, and thus it was *highly* difficult to schedule a timely appointment. Years ago I wanted to see her for my initial visit, but instead I had to make an appointment with Michelle to avoid a three-month wait. I liked

Michelle so much that there wasn't a need to see Dr. F. That was about to change.

There are moments in your life when you realize that you are lucky and if a situation had gone another way you may have died. Hopefully, we only have to deal with that one time at most. Never dealing with that type of situation should be our default setting. Unfortunately, sometimes life doesn't get the memo.

Fortunately, Michelle unequivocally invested herself in helping me find out what was going on. Unbeknownst to me, until after my diagnosis, Michelle had read an article on Non-HPV cervical cancer one week before I came in to see her for the fourth time. I arrived at the appointment and told her that the hormone replacement I had been taking for four weeks was in fact making the symptoms worse. Prompted by the small voice inside her head and the article she read she asked, "Have you ever had a vaginal ultrasound?"

I replied, "No, I have not."

This procedure was one of the first of many diagnostic adventures on my journey. Thank God Michelle is the type of woman who listens to her small intuitive voice. I feel incredibly fortunate and grateful to her in a way that escapes precise expression.

She checked the schedule and gave me an appointment a few days later. I was still in the, "I got nothing to worry about," mode. My history of non-HPV tests and normal pap tests had me cozy and snuggled into a false sense of security.

Next stop: vaginal ultrasound. The directions were simple. I was required to drink a liter of water (which felt like twenty gallons) two hours before the procedure; and hold it through morning rush-hour traffic, waiting in the doctor's office, then onto the exam table and into the stirrups. The first portion of the procedure involved an easy over-the-belly ultrasound. No biggie. I've paid for services at day spas that were not as relaxing. The best part of finishing that portion of the process was getting to empty my bladder.

I was so happy about relieving my poor bladder that when it was time for step two I was still caught up in the celebration. When the large and long probe device came into view, the party ended. All I could think of were the many episodes of *X-files* I religiously watched that involved alien abductions and arsenals of probing devices. I could swear that probe aimed at my "naughty bits" appeared in Season 4, Episode 7.

The compassion of the ultrasound technician was so welcomed. It is mind-blowing that people are so good at these types of jobs. As a former career counselor I can tell you I never asked a client if they were good at such a thing.

Going through "the whole cancer thing," I was asked many questions I had never been asked. The technician gazed at her screen and asked me, "Has anyone ever told you that you have a misshapen cervix?" For a split second I didn't know whether to take that as a compliment or just an observation she was making about what makes me, "unique and special."

After a few seconds I answered, "No." It wasn't a normal, "No." It was one of those drawn out for a good six seconds and ends with my voice at the top of its range. This "no" was racked with much more meaning.

One little word, "no" when translated in my head sounded like, "What are you saying to me right now? Are you asking me that for a reason? What are you looking at? Who else has a misshapen cervix? Is that common? When is this over? Did I inherit that little gem without knowing it? Were my German, English, Scandinavian and Scottish ancestors prone to misshapen cervixes? Again, when is this over?!"

All that stuff was swimming around in my head. So when she said she was going to check the doctor's schedule and left the room, numbness came over me. It wasn't the first time numbness had come over me. Funny thing, even when good things happen I tingle in an uncomfortable way. It's not good.

Excitement triggers the fight-or-flight response whether it's a good or a bad thing. My breathing got shallow and I felt a little nauseous; but I'd had the same response when a script I wrote won a film festival. It's just physiologically confusing. I suppose when your body eventually senses something is not a threat it can relax.

The technician came back in the room and said the doctor could see me the next day. No cell in my body could relax. I felt an escalation of sheer terrorized disbelief, not because I didn't have to wait three months for an appointment, but the whole misshapen cervix thing was shaping up to be a potential life-changer.

I was out of that office as quickly as possible, but did pause to observe the office staff taking on a silent, "Oh you poor thing" on my behalf. I walked out numb from the feet up with an overwhelming urge to Google.

The amount of time spent researching your ailments needs to be tightly monitored right out of the gate. I seek information when in crisis. I always have. Being aware of your saturation point is important because there is a tipping point where you may be making things worse. A good indicator of an overload is finding yourself in the corner in the fetal position suffering from exaggerated self-diagnosed maladies that do not exist.

When I got home and raced to the computer, my research skills turned on, up, and focused. I became aware that HPV causes only 85-90 percent of cervical cancers. The vaccines that are in use today do not guard against non-HPV cervical cancer. Everyone needs to be aware of that and avoid falling into a false sense of security just because you got a shot and a lollipop.

The sharp end of all the arrows were pointing more and more toward a cervical cancer diagnosis. I was trying to stay within my cozy little false sense of security attempting to convince myself I was not going to be in that statistical 10-15 percent, at least for the next 24 hours.

I downplayed it as best I could by repeating my mantra, "I don't have to worry about it until I have to worry about it." After all, Christmas was a couple days away and I had shopping to do. A biopsy wasn't on my wish list. However, it was on my, "To Do List" for the following day.

All females of a certain age who have undergone a gynecological exam are familiar with the notion and the discomfort, the pain – okay I said it, involved in the procedure. We endure it in the name of good preventative health. Going into the biopsy procedure I felt okay because I had a point of reference for this type of discomfort. I knew it was necessary to determine once and for all what was going on in my reproductive organs.

I guess Dr. F had to bring the big guns out for the biopsy. Big guns and a big sample-taking device that felt like a staple remover that rendered a hurt more intense than any previous gynecological exam. This was not exactly a fun way to meet my doctor for the first time. With the grabbing of tissue came more pain and then the "TINK, TINK" sound of the metal instrument hitting the side of the specimen pan. I wondered what the hell was happening down there. I couldn't see what was going on, but then again I didn't want to.

After about eight samples accompanied by eight apologies from the doctor regarding the pain, the process was over. My inside voice said, "Why in the hell would something that painful not be accompanied by some kind of pain control?" Before my outside voice could ask the question, Dr. F told me the results, unfortunately, would take about a week; and she was sorry that I would not know until after Christmas. Put that in your stocking! No, she didn't say that part. However, I did feel like I was at the ending of the worst-ever re-boot version of, *Twas the Night Before Christmas*:

…With a wish and a flare she dashed out of sight…

8

...leaving me stunned and bloody until later that night.

I have always loved Christmas and have had to fight off the negativity of some family members who are haunted by the ghosts of Christmases past. Was I headed into that domain? Was Christmas going to be ruined for me once and for all? I knew the Holidays were getting very, very serious and nothing had turned into something.

"Live Life To Write About It." – Anne Kruse

CH 2 - DIAGNOSIS: DO YOU REALLY WANT TO KNOW?

Most of us are keenly aware of our exact location when we heard the news of an impactful event. I was camping at San Clemente State Beach in California when Elvis Presley died. I was in my bedroom watching T.V. getting ready to go to a college class when I witnessed the space shuttle explode. I was just coming back from walking my dog, Takota, when I turned on Good Morning America to see the first plane hit the World Trade Center. I watched the world as I knew it change when the second plane hit that second tower. The phone rang and I answered it, which if you know me is a rare thing. It was my very dear friend, Sandra, who was living in New York at the time. Together, three-thousand miles away from each other, we watched the first tower collapse. She rushed off the phone knowing that our transmission would likely be cut-off any second. Thankfully, she was escaping to a friend's house in Connecticut where she would be safe. When I walked outside that day all the colors looked different to me. This had never happened to me before, ever. Life was different now for me and for everyone.

Where was I when the news came that I had cancer? December 29th, 2011 is a day that did not start like any other. I had been in limbo for a week waiting for the results of my biopsy. When the first thought of the day creeping into your sleepy brain reminds you that fate is especially uncertain, you definitely want to go back to sleep. Limbo was an odd position to be in. I didn't want to tell too many people about the situation because I didn't know what was going to happen. In fact, the fewer people who knew, the better. On one hand I wanted to do things that distracted me from my situation. On the other hand, when I got distracted from my reality, it was staggering when I suddenly remembered what was going on. Feelings of extreme dread would gush in and crowd out any positive thoughts that may have entered my mind. I gave up trying to have a good Christmas. It worked best for me to keep the reality of my situation in-mind the entire time. I practiced my best version of guarded optimism, until the phone rang.

I'm fortunate to have a detached work/writing studio at home that I lovingly refer to as "The Ranchita." It allows for a quiet work environment free of intrusions from my dog and cat. It was a Thursday. The phone rang and I saw on the caller ID it was Dr. F. My heart sank, my tongue went numb, and my arms went tingly. Interestingly, those can be symptoms of a stroke or when the people from the Publisher's Clearing House Give-away show up at your door with a gigantic check declaring you a Million Dollars Winner. My physiology was once again confused.

"Hello, this is Anne," I said and then listened for an instance of silence knowing that whatever I'm going to hear in this upcoming moment will either be really good or really bad.

My doctor's voice was very assertive yet calm, which slightly threw me into thinking she was going to tell me it wasn't cancer. Don't let voice tones fool you. She said, "Anne, we got the results back and it is cancer. A well-defined mass is on the back side of your cervix. That's why it has gone so long undetected. It is very curable and you are likely looking at a radical hysterectomy and probably radiation, but no chemotherapy. I will be referring you to a nationally-recognized gynecological oncologist, Dr. T. He operates using a robotic technique, and is the top in his field. His office will be calling you to set up an appointment for a consultation as soon as possible. I'm sorry this isn't good news, but you will be in good hands. I work with him a lot, and I will continue to stay up-to-date on your case as time goes by."

We shared a bit of small talk and then the conversation was over; but the journey was just beginning.

At first blush when I read what I just wrote, I realize that initially the news sounded bad; but in comparison with how it turned out, it was the utmost in minimization. Plain and simple, getting the diagnosis was pretty easy in comparison to what I ended up having to endure.

My surgery was not robotically performed due to the large size of the mass. Ah yes, a fully open procedure was performed resulting in an eleven inch scar and the end of my bathing suit modeling career. Chemotherapy was added too, which was supposed to be "well-tolerated." NOT!

You could compare the under-selling of my diagnosis to renovating a house. It's always going to be at least 20 percent more "expensive" than you've been told and the project will take much longer than you anticipated. If it had been as simple as it was conveyed to me I don't think I would be writing this book. Perhaps it happened for that reason; but frankly I would have gladly given up writing this book in a swap for an easier passage.

I've always been curious about the first thoughts people have when they are told they have cancer. Mine wasn't about dying or being afraid; that came later. I have always thought I would die from being tripped by my cat, Mr. Bill, who loves to dart into the path of oncoming humans. Honestly, my thoughts went something like this:

Cancer? That figures! I knew I was never going to get my turn at being a screenwriter. Okay, I hear you God. I don't get to do what I've always wanted to do and have been working my butt off to do. It really was too big of a dream to dream after all; but at least I'm not going to die from Alzheimer's. Thank God!

My writing journey has included many roadblocks. This situation drew into question whether the journey was going to permanently end. I felt extremely defeated and sad. An intense grieving process began even before I told anyone. It felt exactly like waiting in line and working my way to the front for eight years; and then when I got there someone tells me, "Sorry, we ran out of time." I was profoundly sad. FYI, I rarely use the word "profoundly" and usually reserve it for big gut-wrenching emotional times. This was one.

I knew it was nearly impossible to get a writing job in the first place. Who would hire a person who may die before they turn in the next re-write? I know what it takes to package a movie script with a writer, director, cast and crew and how few projects get picked up. The notion of someone taking a chance on hiring a person dealing with cancer just pushed my chances to zero. That's the reality of the situation. Welcome to Hollywood.

Like the lyrics from The Eagles' song *Wasted Time* say, "I'm afraid it's all been wasted time." This never felt more emphatically true. Luckily, these feelings and perspectives evolved, and continue to evolve.

My initial thoughts and feelings were a bit surprising to me. I felt a calm come over me rather than the expected fight-or-flight response. The best word to describe the feeling I was having is: resolved – marked by firm determination; bold, steady; having fixity of purpose. Someone told me that feeling resolve is attributed to clearly knowing who the opponent is, which allows you to focus all your attention. So many times in life when the opponent is imaginary it is usually a result of anxious provocation. Cancer is a real and formidable opponent.

I spend a lot of time lingering in the fight-or-flight response airspace; so when that was absent, I was a bit confused. I knew I would be a compliant patient and would do what I needed to do to help myself. Oddly, it didn't feel like my fight response was being summoned; but unquestionably I needed to come up with a plan of action. If I was going to be caught up in the sea of cancer, I could not fight the tide; but I could build a boat and navigate to a safe shore - destination unknown.

Picture 1: The notes I doodled when talking to my doctor while being told I had cancer.

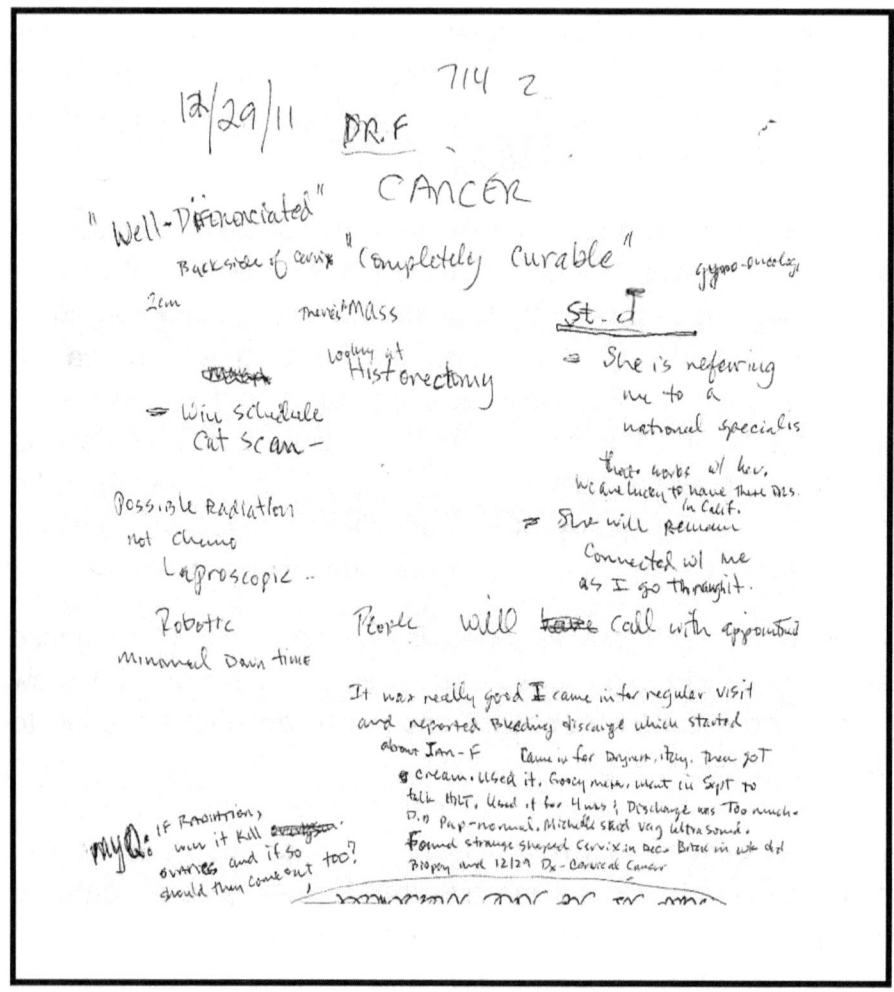

Ch 3 - EXTRA, EXTRA – ANNE'S GOT CANCER

A simple push on the "End Call" button of my phone and my life had changed. Here I was sitting on a secret *and* a cancerous powder keg. I took a few minutes to gather myself, stood up and stepped outside. It happened again, just like after 9/11/01. All the colors outside looked different to me. The vibrancy faded into pale monochrome. I'm a very visual person so I noticed it right away. I don't know what the body is doing when this happens. Recognizing the look and feel of it shifted me into a very different mode.

I was about to ruin a few people's day knowing I had to tell my friends and family what was happening in my life. It was a big responsibility because in one conversation I sent each person on a journey of their own. It was the season for giving, but this little gift was one everyone would return for a refund if they had the chance.

First, I had to tell my partner, Barb. She was my biggest concern because she had been the main caregiver for her father as he suffered and eventually died from mesothelioma caused by asbestos exposure. Also, she and our friend Johnny were already managing a friend's life who had been suffering from early-onset Alzheimer's for eight years. Sadly, Bob, their friend passed away in December, 2012.

Handing Barb another caregiving duty was not something I wanted to bestow upon her. She had already endured caring for me when I suffered a severe back injury in 2006 and couldn't walk for three months without being in agony. We made it through that, but I didn't want to do that to her again.

I walked into the house, found Barb in the kitchen, and she said, "Well?"

I said, "It is cancer."

Details were given and an announcement plan was devised. Barb's calm reassurance was welcomed and helped me make sense of things. A list of family and friends to call was made, and she allowed me the space to prepare for the process. I called people on my list and she agreed to call and tell some people too.

Preparing an e-mail to tell others took some time as I needed to calculate the right amount of information, feeling, and optimism. It needed to show I was educating myself, I was approaching things with a calm resolve; and I was going to keep my sense of humor about it. After all, it's one of the best defense mechanisms I own.

Adding to the dread of telling my friends and family was the fact that I kept this secret during the Thanksgiving and Christmas holidays. I don't do well with deceiving others mainly because I cannot stand being deceived. Warning: PLEASE do not throw me a surprise party of any kind. I will likely want to relinquish our friendship, and won't even think about reconnecting with you on Facebook in twenty-five years.

People are interesting when you tell them about life or death things. Some handle it with grace and are comforting. Others struggle with all of it and will say things that are not helpful in the least. I'm sure in their awkwardness they don't realize what they are saying. I had one friend say after surgery, "Well, how does it feel to not be a woman anymore?" She laughed, and was the only one laughing.

When I told another acquaintance that I had cervical cancer and needed to have a radical hysterectomy she said, "Well, you don't really need that stuff anyway. You aren't having kids."

How could anyone think that either of these comments would be appropriate to say to someone in my situation? The answer: sometimes people don't think before words fall out of their mouths; and then they realize it would have been better to just keep quiet. Unfortunately, they may never understand and will continue to say inappropriate things. Last time I checked this was not a virtue.

Additionally, I experienced some instances of bad timing. I was going through the diagnostic process, being invaded by hands and instruments, and felt like I was taking part in alien-abduction experiments. During this same period, I was also reading scripts and writing coverage analysis for an entertainment attorney for whom I occasionally work. A friend sent me a script from a director-friend of hers and asked me to read it to see if any of the attorneys showed interest in helping to get it developed. Thinking it would serve as a good distraction, I agreed. BIG mistake. It was a horror script which involved a group of people abducting women and ritualistically impaling their genitals. I am serious! I was so taken aback that reading the entire script was not accomplished. Later, I asked my friend if she had read it before giving it to me, which she had not. She knew about my cancer predicament and impending surgery; so when I gave her a brief review of the storyline, she was stunned. The fact that the attorney's office I worked for consisted of three female attorneys and a female creative director, the script was rendered not worthy of their time or attention. What compels people to write that stuff? I shudder to know.

You might have surmised by now that I have never liked horror movies. In fact, I was scared for life at the age of six or seven-years-old when I saw a Vincent Price movie called, *Dr. Fibes*. I had nightmares for ten years. Vincent Price's character was a freak that killed people based on the ten plagues. My parents probably thought I would fall asleep at this double feature, but I didn't. Our family of six rarely went out for family events; but when we did it wasn't always a well-suited occasion for me - being the baby of the family.

I continued to tough-it-out through the holidays. Another friend of mine who had been dealing with breast cancer toasted to the New Year saying, "The worst is behind and we have great things to look forward to," I, on the other hand just went into a numb, faux-cheer response. Ringing in the New Year had a definite phony feeling to it, which really bothered me. I don't want to be phony to my friends.

New Year's Eve and Day were filled with the usual viewing of the Rose Parade and college football bowl games. I planned to wait until I saw the gynecological oncologist before telling the rest of the people on my list.

Two days later I found myself in Dr. T's office, the gynecological oncologist. It was the 3rd of January, 2012. It is funny how the last thing on your mind at a time like this is a New Year's resolution. However, I was resolved to just get through the moments of this day.

The appointment was designed for me to meet Dr. T and allow him to assess the situation. He is a national leader in robotic surgery. My gynecologist, Dr. F, advised me that this was the type I was going to have. The words, "minimally invasive" were ones that brought me comfort. Dr. T's assessment would steer things in a different direction.

It was time to get in the stirrups and face reality. The room seemed crowded, probably because it was. There was Barb and I, Dr. T, an assistant, a nurse consultant, and a diminutive female doctor working with Dr. T as part of a fellowship program. I named her, Dr. Dainty Hands. It's hard not to feel like you're in a cruel puppet show with hands disappearing under your gown. I remember the nurse consultant trying to talk in my ear as a distraction, but I'm not easily distracted especially when an orifice is being invaded.

Dr. T's assessment concluded that the tumor, although large, was well-defined and seemed to have clear borders. It was positioned on the back side of my cervix, which made it hard to detect by normal screening methods. He estimated that it had likely been growing for fifteen years. I was astonished, but accepting of that conclusion because it "connected the dots" regarding some seemingly random symptoms that prior ex-gynecologists had tossed aside as "aging." Then he asked the diminutive doctor to reach inside for a feel because she had much smaller hands than he did and she could get much closer to the mass.

I couldn't help but flash to that scene in "Schindler's List" when Liam Neeson saves the children from certain death and yells at the Nazi commander, "They have small hands! How else can we polish the inside of these bomb casings?!" The camera zooms in as Schindler grabs the wee hand of a girl and raises it in the air.

I guess I was trying to mentally escape the situation and resorted to the movies stored in my head. It actually made me kind of chuckle inside - mostly because I was able to find a bit of humor in this absurd situation.

Dr. Dainty Hands confirmed Dr. T's assessment and plans were discussed. There was a steady stream of information to absorb and understand. It was so helpful to have Barb there because she could be an extra set of eyes and ears - especially helpful when all I wanted to do was close my eyes and stick my fingers in my ears.

A PET scan (Positron Emission Tomography) was scheduled rather than a CAT scan (Computer Tomography) to get a more well-defined diagnostic image of the mass. Rounding out the diagnostics would be a chest X-ray and blood work. According to the operating room schedule, I would be having surgery within two to three weeks. Tick-tock.

CH 4 - WHAT'S A GIRL GOTTA DO TO GET GOOD SERVICE?

I love great customer service. That's one thing cancer affords you for all the other uncomfortable things thrown your way. You have the shortest wait times, closest parking, and cream-of-the-crop nurses and doctors. It's like flying first class, having a car service and personal assistants who really care about you.

Within a day I was in the radiology department being admitted for a PET scan. Great effort was taken to make the process a calm one. There were even warm blankets in the prep room. I was injected with a solution that allows greater contrast to identify any and all cancer cells in my body. I was told the cancer cells are attracted to sugar in the contrast solution. That is mind blowing, isn't it? I don't know what that says about eating a lot of sugar; probably nothing positive.

The protocol allowed an hour for the solution to circulate in my body while I cozied-up with my warm blanket and watched a little TV. The technician came and got me and escorted me to the PET scan room. The size of the donut-shaped machine was a tad intimidating and felt a little like, "Star Wars;" but all I had to do was lie down and intermittently hold still while pictures were taken. The tube wasn't too long and claustrophobic; and soothing music was piped in. The hum of the machine actually made it quite relaxing. When it was all over, the technician asked me how I was doing. I said, "It was great. Too bad cancer has to be involved in such a relaxing situation."

Next, I had a chest X-ray and blood drawn - easy-peezy. All I had to do was await results. Yes, there I was again waiting for results; and they came.

The PET scan was a full-body scan from the top of my head down to the middle of my thighs. That sugar in the contrast solution found its way to my cervix and confirmed the presence of a mass measuring 5.5cm x 6cm x 4cm. The mass did not appear to reach the pelvic floor, the bladder or rectum. That was a HUGE relief. There's something about awful things going on in organs that you can't touch or even feel that make you wonder what else your body is doing behind your back.

Apparently, there were some other things going on inside my body. It was discovered that I had a "borderline" dilation in my aorta, and there was "something" present in my liver. The sugar solution didn't gather in the liver so it wasn't cancer; and the plan was to further evaluate it after my cancer surgery and treatment. This made me feel even more like a genetic garbage can. It seemed my body was imploding and I was only in my forties. Heart issues were never something I worried about; and actually, I didn't even remember where my liver was until I checked my anatomy book when I got home. Boy, we really don't know what's going on inside our bodies. It's like the time the light in my refrigerator wasn't going out when the door closed. How can we know that? I didn't know it until one day I opened the refrigerator to see the entire light assembly melted and dripping into the shelves full of food below. I wondered why the milk had been spoiling so quickly. Like the ever-blazing light in the refrigerator, cancer had been growing in my body along with some other painless, symptom-less problems. The PET scan opened the proverbial door.

I had to go to a cardiologist to have him assess my situation to get cleared for surgery. Luckily, my gynecologist called-in a favor and got an appointment for me within a couple of days. They hooked me up and ran an EKG/ECG (Electrocardiogram), which showed normal heart activity. The doctor assured me that "borderline" is just that. It doesn't mean it's bad; and he said some people are born that way.

Many times throughout the journey I would hang my hat on whatever sounded best. The "truth" felt like an abstract concept anyway. I was relieved to be cleared for surgery, and really wanted the cancer OUT of my body ASAP!

Dr. T's office called and wanted me to meet with Dr. Z, the radiological oncologist for a consultation at their facility. I complied. Arriving at the appointment, I saw that this was the finest set-up around: gourmet coffee, cookies and plush, relaxed seating. I soon realized that the "plushier" the department, the more difficult the experience for the patients. My appointment was merely a consultation. What did I have to worry about?

Sitting and waiting in the radiological oncologist's exam room I noticed the "fixins" for a gynecological exam. I said to myself, "Oh, that's not for me. He's not going to need to do that. We already know the tumor is there and I'm going to have surgery."

Dr. Z entered the room, told me he was going to need to do an exam and I unexpectedly verbally lashed out. Oops! I officially had reached my tolerance level. I thought the appointment was merely going to involve discussing options to radiate the mass, and me saying, "No thank you." I was irritated because the last exam in Dr. T's office caused a bloody situation that nearly ruined the exam room furniture. I dealt with the fallout for three to four days. Having just recovered from D. T and Dr. Dainty Hand's excavation, I wasn't up for another round. I submitted to the exam, which still pisses me off as I'm writing this. The doctor found no big surprises, which was good, but I still think it was unnecessary.

I was astonished by the information Dr. Z shared about other options to surgery. He explained a treatment involving hospitalization (across the street) to prepare me for a procedure; then I would go back to the radiology oncology department and he would insert radioactive pellets into the tumor. The pellets would stay in the tumor for an undisclosed period of time before being removed. The process would be done four times over a period of weeks. I asked, "Who the heck would do that option when they can just have surgery?"

He said, "There are some people who want to save their cervix, uterus and ovaries."

Sympathy-sadness came over me for all the women who wanted to have children and had to endure this kind of treatment in order to have a family. Then, happiness came over me because I wasn't that person. His story was something right out of *Dr. Fibes*, which reinforced my disdain for horror movies. I walked out of there knowing I was in the final stretch. One last pre-op appointment to attend and I was set.

Deciphering all the information coming my way was difficult. Again, if at all possible, I suggest having someone with you to be a second set of eyes and ears. Specifically, you must be able to recognize and determine if information given to you is designed to educate you vs. legally galvanize the doctor vs. pacify you vs. positively manipulate you vs. be real, grounded information.

Dr. Dainty Hands met with me initially about a week before surgery in a small office to review paperwork for a pre-op appointment. Dr. Dainty Hands prefaced our discussion by saying she needed to go over some all-inclusive information with me to make sure I knew as much as I could going into surgery. I really appreciated her approach. She disclosed that she became a doctor because her father died at a young age; and it compelled her to go into medicine. A doctor's self-disclosure always wins points in my book.

She told me there was a possibility that when Dr. T got inside (my gut) he may find things that did not appear on the PET scan, and he would need to close me back up. Doesn't that sound horrible? I already knew this was true for any surgery, but it was sad music to my ears. In fact, they told my mom the same thing back in 1978 when she had breast cancer. Dr. Dainty Hands assured me all indications on my PET scan showed what we were dealing with and the probability of it being different was low. I hung my hat on that.

Our meeting concluded with me signing papers allowing my tumor to be donated to a research library for further exploration into non-HPV cervical cancer. The prospect of adding to knowledge about this rare segment (10-15 percent) of cervical cancer was something I found very meaningful. Without research, advances into new and better prevention methods, detection and treatments cannot be realized. I did my part; and it actually felt a bit like I was part of a really cool recycling program. My tumor was not going to end up in a landfill. It's good to be green.

The second part of the pre-op involved Dr. T explaining that due to the size of the tumor he was not going to do the robotic surgery; but rather an open procedure would be done so he could feel the tissue with his hands to ensure the cancer was removed. I was in store for a large incision and a radical hysterectomy that would remove all my reproductive organs. I was shown diagrams of various stages and types of hysterectomies. This was quite shocking. I looked at it as long as I needed to and then looked away. Sometimes you need to just look away.

My mind was focused on getting that cancerous foreign mass out as soon as possible. Let's also remember other happy thoughts: the fact that I would be saying good-bye to my period once and for all was like looking forward to a permanent Hawaiian vacation. Aloha!

CH 5 - I MISSED GRACELAND FOR THIS?

No matter how well-laid the plans, they can always be uprooted. Cancer, unlike anything else, has probably ruined an incredible amount of vacations, birthdays, weddings - you name it. Cancer is a "Party Pooper."

Memphis was calling me to attend a dear friend's 50th birthday celebration that included a visit to Graceland. However, I was caught in a trap... I couldn't walk out...because I had to have surgery, Baby. Come on - you know I had to work Elvis in somehow.

The days leading up to my surgery were filled with angst, and calling people to tell them I had cancer. There was a point where I simply ran out of time to tell some friends; but they eventually found out. My previous experience with surgeries taught me the importance of getting my digestive system ready for the impact of anesthesia, pain meds and stress. Eating good foods, drinking a lot of water, and taking a cleansing dose of fiber, aloe vera juice, and liquid chlorophyll set me right.

Twenty-four hours before surgery I was given instruction on how to prepare my bowel. My intestines had to be clear to avoid any possibility of bacteria getting into my abdominal cavity should my intestine get nicked or snagged. All these procedures and discussions were adding to the disgust I was feeling about my body and the situation in general. I never felt so repulsed about my own body, which I hoped would be temporary. Believe it or not, that's still a challenge.

The diet of the day: clear liquids and lots of laxatives. Up to that point, I never consumed only clear liquids for an entire day. Sure, I had been sick before and hadn't eaten all day, but this was different. I don't do well when I'm hungry; *no one* does well when *I'm hungry.* Deprivation makes me grumpy.

With a healthy dose of fear and coerced respect for bacterial infections, I was inspired to manage my pre-op potions. I took it easy on the laxatives because history told me that my system reacts too well to these things.

My appreciation for beef broth was surprising. If I have to lose a few pounds in the future, I'm going to welcome broth into my diet plan. I closed my eyes and thought of a steak and savored every liquid bite. What do you know? The pre-op prep wasn't as bad as I thought it would be. A brief relief, but nonetheless a welcomed one.

Driving in the pre-dawn hours to the hospital I was very quiet; and I tried to focus on my breathing. Just making sure I remembered to breathe was a challenge. Barb drove as I closed my eyes trying to find a calm resolve about the day ahead.

Our crack-of-dawn arrival to the hospital felt like getting to elementary school too early. I felt awkward that I was there; and I fool-heartedly tried to tell myself that the hospital must be closed so I should just go home.

Barb and I pulled up and got out of the car. I saw my best friend, Laurie, in the lobby. Darn it! The hospital was open. She always arrives early for every occasion. Apparently this time she got there before the guy who unlocks the door, which made me laugh. Leave it to my pal Laurie to lighten the tension of the moment. Her love and support has gotten me through many of life's challenges.

I have to say that Laurie is not only my best friend; she is the *best type* of friend. She shows up when most people would not. At only five feet tall she is the biggest human being when it comes to really showing me she cares. She understands me, which is such a godsend.

Barb, Laurie and I made our way in and sat in the waiting area. When that door leading to the pre-op area opened, I held my breath. However, by this point, I was ready. Bring it on! We were escorted to the pre-op bays where I got dressed down, dressed up, hooked up, and shaved. Whatever the drugs are that allow you to ease into the process are incredibly helpful, and seductive.

As protocol would have it, the anesthesiologist came in to chat with me. I made sure to tell him that I was definitely going to need that shot for the anti-nausea when I woke up. He assured me he would take care of that.

I felt relaxed and accepting when Dr. T came in brimming with quiet confidence. He asked if I got a good night's sleep and I told him that I did. More importantly, I asked him if he did. He had, and we were all set to go.

Something disturbing happened at that point. A new doctor came out (we later named him Dr. Gruff), and introduced himself. He told me he was working with Dr. T as part of the same fellowship in which Dr. Dainty Hands was participating. He proceeded to tell me the same cautionary tales that Dr. Dainty Hands told me regarding the possibility of Dr. T getting inside my gut and finding things were not operable and he would have to close me back up.

First, I thought he had discovered some new information of which I was not aware. Then I got a tad bit angry that he would be telling me this information when I had already been told. It was upsetting to hear this type of information moments before being wheeled into surgery. I cut him off because I didn't want to hear it again. Needless to say, Barb and Laurie were taken aback by Dr. Gruff's words as well; and Laurie was livid on my behalf. God I love that about Laurie. I had all my bases covered when it came to feeling loved and protected with Barb and Laurie at my side, which is a great thing to feel right before surgery.

A patient is trying their best to calm themselves in preparation for surgery. The stress and emotion of the situation are at a tipping point. My thoughts: Please do not tell me information that I've already heard because my fight-or-flight response is ready-at-the-gate and poised to pounce. The fact that Dr. Gruff was a "newbie" doctor and a new member of Dr. T's fellowship was something to consider. However, this should not absolve a trainee from the responsibility of finding out what a patient already knows. Everyone involved must remember a patient is hanging on every word the doctor says.

It was time to say goodbye. The hugs seemed padded with fear and yearning that everything would be okay. Being wheeled down the hallway, I couldn't help but think that those moments feel the same for people who don't make it out alive. The moment is exactly the same. The outcome goes one way or the other. It is a point of contemplation that still captivates me. Laurie told me later that when she saw me being wheeled down the hall she lost it. She cried all the way out to the lobby, to her car, in the car, and all the way to work. She said it was very upsetting to see a friend potentially being wheeled away for the last time. We were all astutely aware of that. Those of us who have been the loved one left standing in the hall know what that feels like.

As I was wheeled into the surgery room, I noticed how much it looked like the service bay at a car repair shop. I was there to have an overhaul, and the medical staff prepped for the job with precision. The ER nurse was quiet and didn't seem very confident, which caused me to worry. The others made up for her. I love people who have that certain quality that allows you to trust them. Call it "healthy confidence" – not to be confused with inflated ego. There wasn't too much time to worry about it. Once I got on the table, they put the breathing mask on my face and asked me what type of music I wanted to be played while I was under. Before I could answer, "Anything but rap," I was gone.

Waking up from a bad dream or a bad night racked with fever, you feel like dirt. Your mouth feels like dirt. You don't even want to open your eyes for fear the light will somehow scorch your retinas and worsen the headache that is building inside your scull. A wave of nausea sloshes in your stomach. Awaking from radical hysterectomy surgery pretty much felt this way.

Additionally, I had to contend with an onslaught of noise coming from the other side of the curtain in my hospital room. I was not in OZ. By noise I mean a room-filling group of people talking over each other. This was simply noise to me, and I'm sensitive to noises. I was previously told in my pre-op appointment I would have my own room, which made matters worse. Waking up to the collective commotion, I quickly started throwing up. Abdominal surgery and throwing up - GREAT combo. So much for that anti-nausea shot the anesthesiologist gave me.

The most important thing to remember was that I made it through surgery. I was on the preferred "other side" and the cancer was out of my body. Dr. T told Barb that the surgery went as planned. The tumor was well-contained and the surrounding area looked healthy - always a point to be celebrated no matter what.

Barb and I had complained our way into a private room by late evening. Unfortunately, just as I had finally gotten to sleep at 4:00 a.m. Dr. T loudly dropped in to see how I was doing. Coincidently his daughter was having an emergency appendectomy in the same hospital and he thought he'd come see how I was doing. That is not normal procedure. In fact, when Dr. Gruff showed up the next day to see how I was doing, I told him about Dr. T's 4:00 a.m. visit. He thought I was under the influence and hallucinating. It wasn't until Dr. T told him he had visited me at the 4 o'clock hour that he believed me, which proves you can't always discount a groggy patient.

Pain and nausea management became the challenges of the next three days. The pain I was having wasn't even related to the surgery site. I had an excruciating headache and an area of skin outside my wound dressing felt like I had second or third degree burns. The skin looked red. From what my hospital director friend, Stacy, tells me, it is typical to have pain where an instrument called a Bovie is positioned on the skin while the doctor cauterizes the incision during surgery. Apparently laying it on the skin electrically grounds the device. No one copped to that, but I have a feeling it was the reason I was having pain. There is a lot of nerve pain when skin is cut; but this was really weird. That pain persisted for over two weeks. On the bright side, it was a great distraction to everything else going on.

Before I knew it, I was up and walking around the hallway like a track star. When rounding the ward at one point, I found myself involuntarily competing with a nurse who was challenged with her own physical disabilities. Sadly, I walked the hall with much less effort than she did. Admittedly, I do have this odd competitive quirk whenever I'm walking or running on a stadium track. However, I would have been ashamed of myself for racing this woman. My mistrusting mind thought my physical therapist somehow planted this nurse just so I would feel stronger about my recovery. If that was the case, it worked. It was a perfect distraction. I worried about her for the rest of the day. She struggled. Poor dear, she probably needed to retire and no one had the heart to tell her.

Most of my nurses were great at their jobs. One nurse in particular, Virginia, sticks out in my mind as the most kind and caring nurse I've ever met. She was the type of person who probably wanted to be a nurse since she was a kid. Her helping spirit and kindness really set her apart from the others. When I was at my worst, she was there to tell me it would get better, and she was right. The first time you're able to get yourself cleaned up after surgery always sends you on the right path. She even gave me three pair of those funky, stretchy underwear to take home as a parting gift. According to her, they were much easier to use than regular underwear when you have to manage the catheter contraption, which I would be towing home. I love people who give good practical tips.

There were other very impressive things that happened at the hospital while I was there. One of my favorites was the way the hospital allowed patients to order food. It was just like room service. Granted, I had to be on soft foods for obvious reasons, but it seemed so smart and wasted much less food. So many times people don't eat the food and it goes to waste, which adds to the cost of health care. I have to applaud the hospital for this practice. The scrambled eggs were great too.

Getting weaned off the IV pain killers was a challenge. That magic button is taken away whether you're ready or not. Personally, it seems I don't absorb the pill-form pain killers or anti-nausea pills very well. The heavy pain killers are too much for me. My body likes to prove that by exercising its right to reject them via the closest exit. I knew in my heart that two ibuprofen would do the trick if I could only get my hands on some. The type of painkiller that worked for me when I had throat surgery was Tylenol and codeine. I suggested this, but it wasn't taken seriously for some reason. If I had to do it over, I would definitely negotiate that deal with fervor during my planning appointments leading up to surgery. It's important and vital to ensure the doctor's Rx order for your best-fit medication is in place before you reach the point of vomiting.

As long as Barb was there to watch over things while I was in the hospital, I felt safe. Personally, I don't have a need for a lot of visitors while I'm in the hospital. No one really likes to be there whether you are the patient or the visitor. It seems I had just the right amount of visitors during my stay. I am forever thankful to those who rallied for my cause, and I greatly appreciate those who were there in spirit too.

The anticipation of getting released made each day ripe with suspense. The usual goals focus on bowel movements, guttural sounds and gaseous releases. I've been associated with all sorts of athletic events and I can tell you that my desire to achieve a bowel movement and get the hell out of the hospital far exceeded any State championship aspirations. I wanted to go home because I wasn't getting the rest I needed at the hospital. Isn't that ironic? It seems to always be that way for me. Hospitals must feel a little bit like prison so you'll be motivated to get out.

With one last IV push of anti-nausea meds for the ride home, I was dressed and discharged, wheeled downstairs and out the door into the fresh air. I've never been happier to get into rush hour traffic than I was that day, even with a catheter and bag in tow.

It's interesting that some unexpected dreams come true along the cancer journey. After seeing the "horror" movie, *It's Wonderful Being a Girl*, in the 5th grade, a movie every girl was forced to watch to learn about the menstrual cycle, I hoped and dreamed for the day my period would go away. Yes, I said horror movie. Frankly, as soon as the lights came up in my elementary school's auditorium, I began my futile attempts to negotiate with God to please, please, please don't give me a period. Although it took over thirty years of negotiating, I finally closed the deal. I was driving away from the hospital and leaving my period behind once and for all. Now *that's* what was wonderful about being a girl that day; that and getting to go home.

CH 6 – HUGE INFLATABLE GORILLA

Huge inflatable gorillas: advertising at its best - (cue the sarcasm). Somehow I know the car dealership just off the freeway didn't plan to be the source of cruel irony. That's what I get for peeking out of one eye as I sit in the passenger seat resting my head on the car door.

Tethered like the blow-up great ape, I was captive in rush-hour traffic intimately tied to a catheter-bag combo designed to catch the excretion of my wounded but healing bladder. Home is where I wanted to be more than ever.

Being in a hospital allows you to really know what your personal preferences are for healing. Some of them don't happen while you're in there. I'm pretty convinced hospitals believe a bit of discomfort serves as an incentive to get out. That's either brilliant or a symptom of bad patient care. You pick what you want to believe.

If you ask anyone in my family, they will tell you that I've always been a fan of all things comfy and cozy. I think it's genetic because my nephew, Mitch, feels the same way. My environment means a lot to me; and I am sensitive to things that disrupt the peace.

Leaving the hospital behind, I knew I could get the rest I needed if I could just get home. I am fortunate to live in a peaceful neighborhood. I am blessed to have a partner who is one of the best caretakers in the world. I'm not just saying that like when people say their baby is, "The cutest baby ever." Barb, by a preponderance of evidence, all standards and practices, and overwhelming public opinion is THE person anyone would want to have care for them in a time of convalescence. Go ahead; ask anyone who knows her.

This is a good place to talk about a question that needs to be asked. Either the pre-op staff needed to ask me, or I needed to bring it up to them. It's a logistics question that could interfere with a person healing. The question is: What side of the bed do you sleep on at home?

If they are sending you home with a catheter, the adhesive hook stuck to your outer thigh/hip region only allows the bag to hang on one side of the bed. I know this because mine was not adhered to the side that would allow me to sleep on my normal side of the bed. It sounds like a small thing, but to a person with back problems and side-sleeping issues it's a big deal.

Getting home and sliding into the soft, cool bed linens of the guest room that had been set up for my recovery, was a tactile welcome like no other. Everything was calm and quiet; and the soft timbre of wind chimes threw an audible pixy dust into the air. I was home and very, very happy, and medicated; and did I say, HAPPY?

I longed for the arrival of that feeling of being perfectly situated. It finally arrived. I was in bed, the dose of drugs had kicked in, and I wanted for nothing. I was exactly where I was supposed to be. The little comfort-boost of that moment was hearing the phrase, "I'll let you rest." The door clicked shut and that's when the real healing began.

Sleeping is so restorative. I'm not one of those people who must prove that I'm the boss of my body. I know that healing takes its own sweet time; and I respect the agenda that is put before me. Besides, when I turned thirty, it seemed my body was developing a mind of its own and had turned on me. I wasn't going to go toe-to-toe with it. Actually, I had become a bit afraid of my body by the time I hit my forties. Things were going on that made absolutely no sense. For example, close to a year I searched for the right mascara. I was getting dark marks under my eyes by the end of the day. Every manufacturer was vehemently cross-examined for a product - water-proof or not - that would not leave hideous smudges. It was bumming my high, let alone my hopes of becoming a Cover Girl. At one point I thought it was because I was laughing too much. The train of logic went like this: My eyes squint when I laugh, then my lower lashes would rub on the skin under my eyes causing these dirty looking smears. Well, I'm not going to stop laughing; and the thought of ever laughing *too much* doesn't even exist in my world.

I finally discovered that it wasn't because the world had somehow missed the mark on a truly smudge-proof mascara formula. The smudges were not smudges at all. They were the new formation of wrinkle-shadowing. I coined that phrase. They weren't yet wrinkles; they were just creeping into being wrinkles. Bottom line: I was wrong and it wasn't going to be the last time. It can shake a person's confidence. Mine was shaken.

Clocking some good sleep time came easy. Our two dogs and one cat were kept out of my healing zone. Nights were made much more restful because we decided to relocate my cat. Mr.

41

Bill was moved into The Ranchita (my detached, well-equipped work/writing studio) for night time slumber. He has a habit of waking everyone up between 3:00 and 4:00 a.m. for no reason other than he's really old and somehow got permanently switched to Eastern Standard Time.

It worked out so well that we made the change permanent; and now he loves going out there. The Ranchita has better insulation than our house; and he's got a heating pad, cozy bed, and plenty of food - a kitty's dream.

Weaning off of the pain meds and onto an over-the-counter pain reliever was fairly easy and very much welcomed. Within a few days the anesthesia side effects were resolving and I was feeling surprisingly well.

It's funny the hallmarks we choose to celebrate. When I injured my back a few years ago I celebrated being able to stand long enough to take a shower, and to survive the four, thirty-second timed beeps of my electric toothbrush. I will never forget those accomplishments.

The return of normal bodily functions was a cause for celebration. Having a bowel movement was just as important as it was when I wanted to get out of the hospital. Coffee was my friend. I would sip a little and couldn't help but hear the words of my dearly departed Grandma Leone saying, "I just need a few sips to get things going, you know." Cheers, to you Grandma. We all welcome the time when we don't have to talk about that anymore. It is a sure sign of healing that I appreciated; and I'm sure the people around me did too.

On a similar note, I tolerated the "pee bag" and tried to focus on its practical applications. It really is a lazy man's dream and a great way to win side bets at Superbowl parties. Obviously I was able to hold my pee the longest of all the party goers that year, even if I could only attend telephonically.

My appetite and strength were returning and I was definitely on the mend. It was necessary to cut a few pairs of sweats up the left leg seam to accommodate the catheter tube and bag. The logistics of changing pants and underwear became an obstacle course at times. A skipped step in the procedure could lead to spillage. Therefore, special attention was always needed.

Upon my release from the hospital, they gave me an additional small bag to strap to my leg when I went out of the house. Forget that. I just went out with the big bag and carried it in a cloth grocery bag. If I'm going to carry my pee around in a bag it's going to be an environmentally friendly one. I have standards. The extent of my big outdoor adventures with bag-in-tow consisted of doctor's appointments. Going out to public places wasn't something I felt comfortable doing.

Going to my first post-op appointment a week after surgery wasn't exactly comfortable either. It's one of those things that are put before you to see if you can do it. Getting myself pulled together to attend the appointment was a chore; but I looked at it as a challenge. I found out while attending the appointment what the real challenge was: I had to keep the catheter for another week.

I was under the impression I would only have it for a week. My mental focus was on making it through that week. Everything was focused on getting to that mark. I was mentally dismantled when I was told it was never the intent to have the catheter removed at the first post-op appointment. I really felt they lied to me even though I know they didn't do it on purpose. When Dr. T told me that my bladder would benefit from another week of healing, I conceded.

The catheter finally came out a week later. Dr. Gruff, the medical assistant and I celebrated the achievement. Dr. Gruff poured a measured amount of water into a cup connected to the tube leading into my bladder. I could feel my bladder fill; and soon the urge was to empty it. Once I did, we high-fived and celebrated right there in the bathroom as we saw that I was able to produce the same amount of liquid that was poured back into my bladder. I know that sounds funky, but it was fascinating to watch. I felt like a science experiment, and I was totally fine with that. Medical devices are so intriguing!

The bathroom party will always be a great moment to remember. It was hilarious even as it was happening. Hey, my tank was a little low on laughter, so I appreciated the fill-up (pun intended).

The pathology report came back with no real surprises other than Dr. T telling me that they removed thirty-eight lymph nodes during the radical hysterectomy. My first question after I gasped was, "How many lymph nodes do we have?!"

Apparently, humans have over fifteen-hundred lymph nodes. The body adjusts to the loss and the filtration function continues. The body is amazing! Cancer had been detected in one of the thirty-eight lymph nodes in addition to the mass on my cervix that was about the size of a small flattened orange.

I had a similar feeling one time my cat went to the vet to get his teeth cleaned. When I picked him up, they told me - and showed me - that Mr. Bill had to have nine teeth removed. Holy crap! How many teeth do cats have? Poor Bill-the-Kitty. All he had left were those tiny little teeth in front and three canines, which he has since lost. Worry not. Cats adjust well to having no teeth. He still eats dry food, wet food and treats, and can't get enough of them.

Comparing tumors to different types of fruit is a curious practice. I had a benign tumor removed from my thyroid in 2008, which was the size of a small tangerine. In both cases the doctors chose fruits grown in California. I've got to ask: Do doctors in other states use different fruits, or vegetables? Anyway, having that cancerous serving of fruit removed from my body was a relief; and getting surgery behind me was an indicator I was making progress.

Initially, my recovery time was estimated to be four to six weeks. I was really moving along and getting stronger. I was proud of my efforts to do the right things to enhance my recovery. My body was responding well, but chemotherapy was fast approaching. I wondered if there was any chance I could float away on that big inflatable gorilla.

"Live Life To Write About It." – Anne Kruse

CH 7 - READY FOR NOTHING

There are some days in my personal history that stick out more than others. March 10, 2012 was not a good day. Bottom line: I had a horrible experience in the radiation therapy center during my mapping appointment prior to commencing radiation treatments. The appointment involved getting a mold made of my body that was used to keep my body still during radiation treatments. Also, the medical technicians determine other factors and "map" a plan for directing radiation toward the targeted areas of my body. This is the appointment during which I got a few tattoos, without the use of any liquid courage.

Let's get right to it. You may want to plug your ears. During my mapping appointment I had to lie perfectly still on a table with a tube inserted into my rectum that was shooting in contrast solution. Additionally, a five-inch wooden swab was placed in my vagina, and an IV was in my arm to infuse more contrast solution. If that doesn't sound like an alien abduction experiment, I don't know what does.

Dr. D, was my radiology oncologist rather than the doctor I met prior to surgery. I opted to do my radiation at a facility closer to my home. Her nurse, Agnes, did not demonstrate a confident demeanor. Consequently she fumbled with various parts of the procedure. Everything she said, and the way she acted made me think it was her first time doing the procedure. Perhaps she was filling-in for someone who never made it back from lunch. She kept apologizing over and over to the point of annoyance.

The male technician stepped out of the room to take a scan of me. Then it was Agnes' turn to push the IV and exit the room. Unfortunately, when Agnes mishandled the tubes leading to my arm, she nervously pushed the IV and the fluid exploded out of the tube and all over my face, neck and chest!

Instead of attending to me, she RAN OUT of the room screaming the male technician's name leaving me absolutely helpless. I was left thinking that the fluid all over my face, neck and chest was radioactive, and I was majorly screwed. Having items stuck into my orifices and being forced to lie absolutely still was hard enough. When Agnes exploded radioactive solution in my face then ran out of the room screaming and slammed the door behind her, sheer panic and extreme anger took over my body. I was yelling but no one was listening.

Agnes finally re-entered the room and explained that she ran out because they needed to get the picture taken immediately. They only had a short amount of time to work with the contrast solution. I perceived this as Agnes choosing *her performance* over my *well-being* because she was afraid that Dr. D would get mad at her.

I was livid and told her so with a few expletives peppered throughout. That's another thing: during my journey I cussed more at doctor's offices and during medical incidents than any other time in my life. They aren't proud moments, but I got pushed to points far exceeding my expectations. I could only take so much before my polite manners found their devilish twin, and all hell broke loose.

Later, Dr. D entered the room to calm my concerns and advised me that the contrast solution was not radioactive. I wanted to believe her, but I didn't. I was in paramilitary mode and I trusted no one at this point. All the while Agnes was in the background nervously repeating what she had done, trying to explain away her wrongdoing.

I swear if she was going to apologize one more time I was going to get physical, and actually told her, "You need to stop apologizing right now because you are really pissing me off."

To that she said, "I'm sorry."

I hated doing it, but I had to "shush" her.

I got off that table as fast as I could and was ready to literally hit Agnes in the face. I didn't care that I towered over her. It would have been quite a scene. What she did to me was unforgivable, and certainly unforgettable. As a result, I had to undergo treatment for PTSD-like symptoms. In the event of any type of recurrence, I will not be going back to that radiology oncology center. It is extremely unfortunate because I really like Dr. D; but a doctor is only as good as her staff. Her nurse did not demonstrate the essential skills and abilities to make me feel comfortable. Agnes needs a warning label.

I left the office with a bad attitude and three tattoos to mark the spots for radiation treatments: a period-like dot on the side of my right hip, a dot on the side of my left hip, and a dot about four inches below my belly button. I'm not a fan of tattoos. I've never really felt passionate about something to the level that would warrant a lifetime display on my skin. I have freckles and they're enough to deal with during my lifetime.

Extreme disappointment came over me when I realized my new tattoos looked like periods. I had finally gotten rid of my period at the hospital during surgery, and now it was back in tattoo form forever. (Cue the rim shot) Thank you, I'll be here all book.

Did the fiascos at my mapping appointment make me gun-shy of medically related events? Yes. I now enter any procedure using my relaxation techniques and visualizing a successful outcome. If needed, I have my own panic button to hit when I feel the process is not going well. Usually, it revolves around my sense of the person's abilities, which may or may not trigger foul language. I have to advocate for my own healthcare and the cancer-chemo-radiation journey taught me well.

Three days later, March 13, 2012, was another one of those days. It started out okay. I was six weeks post-surgery and feeling pretty good. I felt that I was healing nicely and bouncing back; but I had no idea the toughest part of the process was still ahead. If my cancer journey had ended after surgery alone, I would have marched on with life without writing this book.

Chemotherapy and radiation were approaching more quickly than I thought. One of the first things my chemo oncologist, Dr. P wanted me to do was attend a, "Chemo Class." I'm certain what knowledge I gained from that experience was not what the directors of the program intended for me to learn.

Research shows that giving information to people who are in an uncertain situation will alleviate, or at least help manage the stress and anxiety individuals are feeling. I can tell you, based on my empirically derived research, when information is given in a disorganized, haphazard, convoluted and unclear manner, the opposite occurs.

I'll set the scene for you as if it were a scene in a movie script:

FADE IN:

INTERIOR – LARGE CONFERENCE ROOM – DAY

Florescent lights glare on the grease-shined face of one seemingly nervous female instructor (20's).

Scattered throughout the room were attendees: a cute older couple with matching cardigans; a heavy-set woman in a wheelchair sitting beside her very skinny husband; and three women - likely sisters.

Barb and I rounded out the cast of characters; all of us were not real happy to be there.

FADE OUT:

I was already feeling on-guard before entering the building due to my experience at the mapping appointment. When it came time to start the "class" and the Power Point presentation took a dump, I wasn't surprised. Murphy's Law was thematically weaving its way through my week.

The audio-visual guy (AV guy) tried to fix the projector device, but time was ticking. I could feel the anxiety building in the room. Judged on the eye-rolling I shared with my fellow classmates, it was bubbling inside them as well.

For forty-five minutes the AV guy tried to fix the projector while the instructor nervously ran rough-shot through some hand-outs about chemotherapy. It didn't seem to bother her that everyone could barely understand what she was saying. She came across as scatter-brained and insensitive. Perhaps she had become too dependent on the Power Point presentation. When it failed, she lost her way.

At one point she asked each of us what type of chemo we were having. As each person told her what chemical was going to be coursing through his or her veins in the very near future she yelled out, "You lose your hair!" and moved to the next person.

By the third person she didn't even wait for the person to complete the pronunciation of the chemical before she yelled out, "You lose your hair!" When she got to me, I told her I already knew that Cisplatin didn't cause my hair to fall out.

I was getting so pissed off at her and felt protective towards the elderly lady in the room. I've got a soft spot for the elderly. She had a perfect little hairdo; one that she's probably had for the last thirty years and gets done by the same hair dresser every Tuesday. Chemo was going to send it bye-bye, which made me very sad. The instructor's behaviors demonstrated to everyone that she was not in-tune with her audience's feelings. It really was illogical that the department put an employee in charge that clearly lacked the aptitude and abilities for such an assignment. We can't blame it all on the Power Point failure.

Side Note: The reason why people lose their hair during some chemo treatments is because the chemical is targeted at the fastest growing cells, which many times are the cancer cells. Ironically, I did NOT learn that in "Chemo Class." The chemo targets those fast-growers and subsequently other fast-growing cells in the body die or get really inflamed. The fastest growing cells in the body are hair cells, and mucus membranes (mouth, intestines, eyes etc.).

The fastest healing cells are the fastest growing cells. It all made sense once I figured this out. I was lucky. I didn't lose my hair. Instead, I decided to let mine grow in hopes of donating it to "Locks of Love" who produce wigs for cancer patients and others who lose their hair. However, a friend told me that you can't donate hair that is colored, which ruined my plan. I'm going to keep hiding the gray for now; but I did decide to let my hair grow, just because I could.

One thing that greatly worried me was that my pets were going to be exposed to me after I was exposed to deadly chemicals and radiation. When my beloved dog, Takota, was dealing with cancer before he passed away I read about chemotherapy for pets, which I did not put him through. Great caution was to be taken when handling any waste products or bodily fluids because of the exposure to the deadly chemotherapy chemicals. If I had been warned about pet-chemo-fallout, would I need to take precautions to ensure my pets were not being exposed to my fallout?

I said to the instructor, "I'm concerned about my pets."

The instructor responded, "You don't have to worry. Your pets won't hurt you."

I wasn't worried that my pets would harm me. It was the other way around. That was 100 percent non-responsive to my question. I didn't even bother commenting. I was perplexed and so was everyone else. It was a lost cause at that point.

Once the disturbing introduction of "Chemo Class" was finished, we were taken on the next phase which involved a tour of The Chemotherapy Infusion Center. For the record, I've been in those horror-filled Halloween mazes where half-eaten monsters scare the living crap out of you. The idea of going into The Infusion Center may elicit the same adrenaline-charged fight-or-flight response. Just be prepared.

The anticipation was actually worse than the reality. For all intent purposes, it looked like a beauty salon with lounging chairs and T.V.s at every station. I'm sensitive to the vibe of my surroundings and this infusion room wasn't so bad. If I let my mind linger on what goes on in there and start to worry about everyone's struggle, then I have a problem. It seemed like it would be okay, tolerable. I could do it.

It was a Tuesday and I was mentally preparing to start my chemo the next week just as my oncologist had indicated. Barb and I planned a weekend getaway before starting the chemo and radiation journey. My goal was to ease into it and take it in stride. I was proud of my plan. It seemed so level-headed and calming.

I was standing there mid-thought when I heard a woman say, "Is there an Anne Kruse here?"

I perked up thinking I left something behind in the classroom, like my hope to learn something. I smiled and responded, "Yes, I'm Anne Kruse."

She replied, "You're starting chemo tomorrow. So be here at 7:30 and you will be here for eight hours. You can bring food if you like."

My smile wilted and I was stunned into silence. I looked at Barb and she didn't know what to say. I was already pretty emotionally detached due to the experiences of the previous few days; so I really didn't feel anything other than a numb buzzing sensation.

I used to work at a company where on occasion someone would have a mundane task thrown upon them and he or she would practically explode. Try getting chemo sprung on you when you're not ready for it. You WILL have a new perspective when it comes to the petty things in life. What do you know? I guess I did learn something from "Chemo Class" after all.

"Live Life To Write About It." – Anne Kruse

CH 8 - YOU DON'T KNOW WHAT YOU DON'T KNOW

There are plenty of times when we use our prior experience to get us through a difficult situation. We can access our acquired skills and use them, which is one of the best advantages to growing up. However, when experiencing something for the first time you don't have a point of reference upon which to draw confidence and self-assurance. Who gets chemicals shot through his or her veins and radiated by a huge machine until you do? You don't know what to be afraid of, and what not to be.

My "rule of thumb" as I entered the chemo and radiation phase of my journey was to trust no one, and pay attention to what people were doing. I could not expect people to always do their jobs. I know that may sound critical; but who better to be a supervisor over my services than me? It also seemed a little paranoid, which I'm certain is a by-product of the entire journey.

The human body is fascinating how it focuses on surviving. The procedures I was engaging in felt like threats to my survival rather than efforts to help me survive. I'm not surprised I became increasingly paranoid and critical as time went on. Negative experiences were triggering primal responses.

Some people don't stick up for themselves, especially in a medical situation. I can harness "the crazy" if I need to make a point. I'm agreeable and cooperate for the most part. If I have questions, I am not afraid to ask them. However, this whole process had me off-balance and I was definitely not at my best – far from it.

My chemotherapy and radiation schedule was set. I would have radiation treatments five days a week in the afternoons for six weeks. I would simultaneously have chemotherapy every Wednesday for eight hours. Wednesdays were the toughest days because I had to endure eight hours of chemotherapy followed by radiation. It is easy to write about the logistics of the schedule; but it is difficult to be reminded of the relentless and crippling nausea that I felt, which I will detail later.

A plan was arranged for me to start my chemotherapy and radiation on the same day. I had to be at The Infusion Center by 7:30 a.m. for chemotherapy. The eight-hour long chemo sessions consisted of blood work, two hours of IV hydration followed by forty-five minutes or so of anti-nausea and steroid IV, followed by two hours of chemotherapy comprised of Cisplatin (a platinum (heavy metal) based drug) followed by two hours of IV hydration again. Cisplatin is known to be very hard on the kidneys and thus hydration was essential to a successful and less-damaging infusion treatment.

The first day Barb and I arrived to find the waiting room at The Infusion Center packed with sick people trying to get well. It was in that moment I realized cancer knows no boundaries. I had been warned to focus on myself because everyone's story can overwhelm your already overloaded psyche.

It's hard not to compare yourself to others in the room. Having a background as a counselor, AKA Professional Listener, it was even harder not to listen to a man talking about his wife who was sitting next to him. His wife was experiencing her eighth recurrence of cancer, and thus her eighth time doing chemotherapy. He was doing all the talking as she sat there staring off into space. It was touching to see how much he cared for her; but I couldn't help wonder if she was tired and didn't want to do it anymore. On one hand it was touching. On the other hand it was horrifying.

Here I was sitting in my jammies with my lunch cooler waiting to have my first session listening to this very emotional conversation. I had to lean over and put my elbows on my knees, looked at the ground and stuck my fingers in my ears so I wouldn't have to listen to it anymore - hey, whatever works. Luckily, within a couple of minutes I was called back into the infusion room for my treatment.

We were lead past twenty or so chemo lounges (AKA the really comfortable pedicure spa chairs). I can tell you no one was getting a flower painted on their big toenail that day.

When we arrived at a private room toward the back of The Infusion Center, I was somewhat impressed. They told me I would have a private room with its own bathroom because I would be there for so long. That sounded like special treatment, which unfortunately made me leery. Now, if it was a hotel, spa, or something fun like that, this type of treatment would be fantastic. I was scheduled for eight hours, but at least the amenities were great.

I entered the room trying my best to remain optimistic even though ambivalence had taken over my state of mind. The area seemed comfortable and clean. They assigned me a nurse, Norma. She was the quintessential old-school, been-around-the-block kind of nurse. I was so relieved. She had a dry sense of humor and she had that seen-everything wisdom that helped her take command of the situation. I appreciated her confidence and demeanor. She was calm, and that helped me remain calm - that is until her assistant came in the room.

To my astonishment there standing before me with the assignment to start my first IV bag of hydration was the women who "taught" the "Chemo Class" the night before. Norma assured me "Chemo-Class Gal" (CCG) was simply going to start the IV and that she (Norma) would be taking care of me all day. I went along with it and CCG started my IV. She set the timers, checked the IV lines and left the room.

I found out that all the nurses and assistants in the infusion center are forced to take turns "teaching" the "Chemo Class." This is a practice that should be revisited based on my class' experience. Regardless of faulty audio-visual equipment, not everyone is a teacher, and every student knows it.

When Norma checked on me about twenty minutes later, she asked me how I was doing. I told her my arm was burning really bad. She said that was because I was nervous. My arm never burned before when I was nervous in any other situation, I can assure you. I wanted to believe her, so I just endured the pain. Of course that was the wrong thing to do.

Norma checked on me again and my arm had started to show a trail of blood under my skin. When Norma saw it she exclaimed, "How come you didn't say anything?"

I said, "I did say something and you said it was because I was nervous."

It took about six weeks for my arm to heal from that first introduction into my vein. Needless to say, after that CCG was black-balled from starting IVs. I guess you take one for the team sometimes whether you were even aware you were on a team.

The bright spot of my days in chemo was this couple who volunteered at The Infusion Center handing out graham crackers, juice and blankets. They made me smile every time I saw them. The woman looked like a character the late, great comedian, Gilda Radner, used to play on *Saturday Night Live,* named, Judy Miller. The woman was flat-chested and wore white overalls and was really skinny like Gilda. I loved Gilda Radner; so this woman already had me in her corner. She was a little dorky in the most kind and generous way. She was a dear, dear person; and you could tell that she absolutely loved her husband.

Her hubby seemed a little bit "along for the ride"; but he was considerate and attentive. The big ponytail hanging down the middle of his back was well-groomed, and spoke to his cool-hippy-vibe. He was my connection for apple juice and anything I wanted. They had been volunteering for two years and loved it. They were my angels. It was obvious their goodwill made a huge difference to a lot of people in that room. I made sure I told them how much I appreciated them. What a great couple.

I really didn't know what to expect in terms of eating and drinking during my eight hour stay. Most people's references, mine included, are from television or movies; and goodness knows those are exaggerated for dramatic impact and always have commercial breaks. I was told to pack a lunch, so I did. Interestingly enough, I was able to eat while I was there. I learned that the ONLY place I did not feel nauseous was when I was in the chemo chair because the anti-nausea drugs in my IV were going straight into my system. When not in The Infusion Center, I took the medication in pill form that had to travel all the way through my stomach to be absorbed. It never worked well.

For that reason, I actually, and very surprisingly, looked forward to Wednesdays. It was my only break from the relentless 24/7 nausea that absolutely crippled me, my outlook, and everything for six long horrible weeks. My nausea has its own chapter - Chapter 13 - for how unlucky I felt. It was the absolute worst part of my entire journey; and I mean that with every bit of sincerity I can muster.

During a typical infusion session I saw many people come and go as I sat there for eight hours. Some people would be there for forty-five minutes, others two hours, and still others for four. I wondered about everyone's story (not in a "nosey" way). I love a good story. Some men would come in, say nothing, get hooked up to an IV, do their time, and leave. A few women would bring two visitors and talked the entire time.

The cutest therapy dog, Reggie, was a great distraction for us during infusion. He was a spaniel with back and brown spots, and had a willingness to make everyone his friend. There was no shyness or apprehension toward meeting anyone as he gently crawled into your lap. What a great service dog. His momma was so proud.

I watched a lot of TV while I was there. Multiple episodes of, *The King of Queens*, were always on the air. I have not seen an episode since finishing chemotherapy.

Witnessing a couple of people having really bad reactions to their chemo drugs was unnerving. It was never comforting to see paramedics and doctors running across a room attending to a person screaming for help. How do you buffer yourself from that? Answer: I didn't. It was like sitting in a horror movie; and by now I think I have made it very clear - I hate horror movies!

Additionally, the presence of extremely toxic chemicals in the room was never a soothing feeling. Waste was disposed in a special bin with warning labels plastered on the side. It felt like I needed a, "Silkwood Shower" every time I left. For those of you who don't understand that reference, it's from the movie, *Silkwood*. Meryl Streep played Karen Silkwood, a whistle-blower who worked in a nuclear power plant. She was intentionally exposed to fallout. In one scene, the men in their hazmat suits forcibly scrubbed her down in the shower. Great movie - harsh shower - poor Meryl.

Each infusion session involved a different nurse, and interestingly enough my favorite was, Nurse Jackie, which is one of my favorite TV shows. There was also a Nurse Navigator, the Rock Stars of the nursing staff, who made sure others were doing their job. She was so helpful with realistic tips about natural alternatives for nausea; and she was the first person who had any information about the use of medicinal marijuana.

I was fortunate to have another Nurse Navigator, Colleen, at The Cancer Prevention and Treatment Center located a few miles away from The Infusion Center. She was, and still is, the greatest link I had and continue to have through the entire cancer experience. Now, when I see her it's like seeing an old friend. She is a top performer and I was lucky to benefit from her aspirations. She is the entire package: caring, kind, smart, thorough, and she *remembers me.*

I tried to stay open-minded about each person during the progression of my treatment. Some made it very difficult. A certain Nurse Practitioner, Cathy, would come in and say things like, "Well how's the patient doing who's the only one that gets nauseous with radiation?"

This was not, and never will be helpful to say to someone struggling with REAL, not imagined nausea. That's one thing about going through this course of treatment: you will likely be forced to deal with someone who has never been through chemo or radiation telling *you* how *you* feel. The last thing a cancer patient, or any patient for that matter, needs to hear or feel is that they are crazy. I was poo-pooed by a few doctors over the years about my health concerns; and low and behold it ended up being cancer. Even my radiology oncologist confirmed that plenty of people get nauseous while going through radiation. I told Cathy what Dr. D had said, but she continued to imply that she doubted my sickness. It was bizarre. I finally had to ask her to please stop.

My schedule of chemo and radiation moved along; and my fight response got weaker and weaker. It was difficult to simply get through the day. To hear someone say crap to me under normal circumstances would have rallied my inner-warrior princess; but in my condition it actually made me feel even weaker. Right now as I'm writing this, I fantasize about going over to the building where she works and confronting Cathy. It's one thing for her to do it to me, but I have a huge protective response for others. If she is minimizing me, who else is she hurting with her "helpful" comments? Maybe she thought she was being funny. Someone told me a long time ago that humor should never be put in the hands of amateurs.

Six weeks of chemotherapy left my veins bruised, bumpy and tattered. For whatever reason, my chemo oncologist did not suggest having a port implanted to receive chemotherapy. Consequently, when I went in for treatment the nurses had to find a really good vein – six times. By my last session, I could feel lumps along the veins running down both my arms. This took a good six months to heal. No one tells you about that. It did give me insight into those who are addicted to inter-venous drugs, and how damaged their systems must be.

Other than having a glorious break from relentless nausea, Wednesdays were tougher than any other day. Two hours before the end of my infusion session I had to start forcing myself to drink water so my bladder would be full during my radiation treatment. It was crucial that my bladder be full of liquid to protect it from being damaged by the radiation rays shooting at a body part called the "vaginal apex." That sounds like a place where the TSA searches you before going on a flight. I was told it is the point at which the organs, including the cervix, uterus and ovaries were removed.

Forcing myself to drink water meant I would eventually have to fight the urge to release it, which is always uncomfortable. I did this five days a week. Every day, but Wednesday, I would be incredibly nauseous and have to force down two, sixteen ounce bottles of water. Then I had to hold it until my radiation treatment was done. If you've ever been stuck in traffic or somewhere and had to hold your pee, when you finally get over the toilet it is one of life's greatest feelings of relief. Imagine doing that for six weeks. Can you relate? Probably not. It really is much worse than you can probably imagine.

Initially, my radiation appointments were scheduled for 10:00am. I could not function at that time so I requested they be moved to 3:30pm; and I still had a hard time getting there. Living five minutes away from the treatment center made it possible. Here I was holding what felt like gallons of pee, and stifling dry heaves as Barb dropped me off in front of the building. As I walked toward the building, I always kept an eye on the bushes along my path in case I had to hurl.

Once inside The Radiation Center, I walked straight to the dressing area where I would change into a gown and put my clothes into a locker. This is where I would see other female patients in the private waiting area. We would say hello to each other and chat on occasion while the Dr. Phil show droned on in the background.

I met a lady who was having a recurrence of breast cancer, which she had seven years prior. This was her third recurrence. Additionally, her brother was dealing with his own recurrence. Despite her predicament, and a wildly irritated rash on the skin surrounding the chemo port in her upper chest, she demonstrated true strength and a positive attitude. She was impressive.

Another woman lived in northern California and came down to southern California to stay with her son. He thought she would get better treatment. She had a colorful hat to cover her bald little head, and bright red lipstick that likely helped her feel more like a lady. Cancer really does a number on that whole concept.

The chats I had with these women while sitting in a white gown made me think about heaven's waiting room. It reminded me of the movie, *Defending Your Life*, with Meryl Streep and Albert Brooks. Yes, another Meryl reference. I highly recommend watching this movie if you go through a life-or-death situation. I had seen the movie before, but this time I saw it through completely different eyes. They were still my eyes, but the way I looked at life had dramatically changed. Spoiler alert: Albert Brooks' character has to defend his life and answer to the courts in heaven as to why he let fear operate so heavily throughout his life. It held him back from living, which didn't make God very happy.

The radiation technicians at The Center were great. Each session would only take about five minutes. I would enter the big room with the huge radiation machine, and they would ask me to identify the picture of myself on a screen hanging on the wall. I guess you don't want to juice the wrong person. They would also ask me if the music was okay or if I wanted it changed. That was a nice touch.

Once I was identified and happy with the music, I would lay down on the table positioning myself in the mold/form we made during my horrendous mapping appointment. It held my lower body and legs in place. I put my hands above my head and tried to relax. The two technicians would move my body to line up the Sharpie pen-drawn lines and tattooed dots on both my sides, and the one four inches below my belly button. These would match up to markers on the table that ensured an accurate shot of radiation. As I lost weight, the mold/form didn't fit as well; but they always made sure I was in line and ready for the shot, which was their cue to leave the room.

From their radiation-safe room I was told over a speaker system to stay still. Then, the machine would turn on and make a potent wind-aided winding noise. The huge arms of the machine would move over and around me. It always felt a little like I was in the Griffith Park Observatory. Strange reference, but it always seemed like this radiation machine was straight from outer space. It was a bit like the scene in the movie *Gravity* when Sandra Bullock's spaceship first gets hit by an asteroid, or whatever it was. As I recall, she was nauseous throughout her entire journey just like me.

I made it a practice to thank my radiation techs each and every visit. We would all celebrate the countdown after every treatment. Chatting with them for any length of time wasn't possible because I was holding my pee and needed to leave. Just one extra sentence during a visit caused a mishap which had me butt-clenched and scissor-stepping down the hall to the bathroom. Those feelings of relief were always appreciated because they meant the water torture was over and my treatment was one visit closer to being complete.

The technicians thanked me for being so positive during the radiation pilgrimage. I told them I thought I was being rather irritable; but they assured me that I wasn't. Chemo, radiation, and holding my pee made me pretty cranky.

They told me some people were really, really crabby. I said, "It's probably because they're going through all this crap."

One technician assured me that some people are just grouchy and will always be grouchy. They should know.

The song that played during my last session was the Mommas and the Pappas, *Leavin' On A Jet Plane*; and I couldn't have been more excited. As the lyrics played, "Don't know when I'll be back again," I adamantly said out loud, "May that be, NEVER."

We all high-fived once I completed that last radiation session. When I walked out of the building, I knew within a few days I would not be nauseous any more. This was the most exhilarating thought I had in a very long time. Truly, the feeling was better than when I graduated from college with my Bachelor's degree, my Master's degree, and the UCLA film school's screenwriting program combined.

Technicians, Darrell, Jan and the rest of the crew made my visits bearable. We accomplished the goal together. I appreciated them immensely; but in the future I would prefer to only see them outside The Radiation Center. I received a certificate of completion in the mail from the staff. It was a feeling of accomplishment far beyond what I had anticipated.

I often hear people say that people going through cancer surgery and treatment are heroes, and are such an inspiration. I'm going to say this straight up and flat out: I NEVER felt like a hero or an inspiration in any way shape or form. Perhaps this speaks for many other patients too. I felt like a prisoner at every turn. It never got any better until it ended. There is no candy coating on any part of living through cancer.

If people think going through cancer treatment makes you a hero, then prisoners should be seen as heroes too. All your freedoms, dignity, who you are, and what you look like are taken away. I'm pretty sure Marvel has never had a cancer patient as a comic book superhero. "Cancer Girl saves the day!" I'm not buying it. However, I have seen radiation and other toxic accidents cause a character to develop a super power. If that happens to me, I'm sure I'll be writing another book and adapting it for the big screen. I'd go to see that. Wouldn't you?

CH 9 - I'M IN A HEAP AND LIFE'S ON HOLD

One of my first real jobs after graduating from college involved working as a rehabilitation counselor helping high school students with disabilities get connected with school or work programs following graduation. This program was called, The Transition Partnership Project, designed to help these students engage in something productive and to help them avoid "falling out the end of the drainpipe," as we used to say.

When cancer treatment was over, I felt a little bit like I was hanging by my fingernails on the end of a drainpipe, and I was losing my grip. Insurance covered the treatment, but it did not cover everything I had to do, and still do, to recover and rejuvenate my war-battered body.

Why wouldn't insurance cover these things? This is only one of many questions that arose through the cancer journey. A more productive avenue to take was to ask, "What can I do to ensure that I find a way back to good health, stay healthy and set the stage for a future that allows me to thrive?"

The problem is I didn't even know where to start. Luckily, I had been to a few really great doctors and knew some people who had success with traditional and alternative forms of wellness. I know it takes a village. Within that village, I have clear boundaries about some of the available "healing" modalities.

I will listen to anecdotal evidence because if something positive happened to one person in a case study, then I may be the second one to benefit. Closing doors isn't my thing. However, I've seen many health practitioners, doctors, and dentists close themselves off to possibilities because of limited thinking and overactive egos. I, as a patient, need to be aware that accepting everything *one* authority figure tells me may not provide the all-encompassing answers to my questions.

Research classes during my college undergrad and graduate studies were some of my favorites. Researchers know that every scientifically-controlled study starts with an idea that may have stemmed from one person's experience. When I was looking for answers, I simply couldn't shut myself off to any possible truth that may benefit me. Closed minds have ended up in the heads of dead people. That's harsh, but you get my point.

Looking at myself holistically – the mind, body, spirit – I had to address all of it back then, today, and I will continue to do so in the future. My beliefs about so many things had changed. My thinking had to be analyzed, shuffled, and reconstructed. My body had suffered a huge excavation in the creative center of my being; and I felt aghast by what was left behind. Although my spirit felt broken, I knew the source that created me would also heal me. I knew this to be true even though the heavy-clad rope that connected me to my source felt withered to a thread. I was concerned about how long the healing would take.

If life is to go on, then guess what? Management strategies are a requirement. Absolutes are impossible. And depression is omnipresent if you allow it.

I see plenty of books that seem too "happy-shmappy" about recovery and everything that comes with it. I guess I'm a realist. I'm not afraid of having a bad day, week or month because those are real experiences and part of life.

Life is not black or white. Real life is lived in the gray area. I have to stop myself sometimes from trying to find the one and only "truth." I remember going to a seminar and the room was filled with about five-hundred people. They were all seeking their "truth." That was really eye-opening to me. If everyone just keeps looking and wondering, how will they ever find peace? Forcing the notion that you may find the truth about life carries a lot of pressure. There's an Indigo Girl's song titled, "*Closer to Fine*," with a line that says, "The less I seek my source for some definitive, closer I am to fine." It's comforting to know that my mid-90's fan-frenzy for those lesbian-folk singers was not a complete waste of time.

This chapter details that stage, that moment of exhale and the, "Okay then, now what?" It is like that moment when you graduate from college, have no job lined up, and you've got nothing but fear, anxiety and the real world staring at you as you wait to make your next move.

At least when I graduated from college my parents gave me a trip to Hawaii, which gave me a little mental break before diving into my future career. However, on the plane ride home I sat next to a six-year-old girl. We were making kid-based small talk when I told her I had just graduated from college with my bachelor's degree. She looked up at me and asked, "Do you have a job yet?" Why I allowed a six-year-old to impose pressure upon me speaks to the state of mind I was in at the time.

When I graduated from cancer surgery, chemo, and radiation I couldn't afford to celebrate by going to Hawaii, or anywhere for that matter. I rewarded myself with a well-deserved new supply of underwear; and quickly realized that my job was to find a way to move forward with life. After making it successfully through the process I was excited to know that life was taking applications.

Cancer definitely pushed the pause button on my life's recorder. I didn't realize that until I got further away from the initial event. It was a paralysis that caused me to avoid getting invested in anything. It made me feel a bit zombie-like when I think about it.

I'm better now, but in the pre-cancer days when I would make plans for a trip or concert, I never wondered if I was going to be okay when the time came to go to the event. I went to incredibly picturesque Carmel, CA for the first time about a year into my journey. It was also the first time I thought it might be my last time. It was a very strange and upsetting feeling. However, it forced me to develop a new perspective. Now, I focus on appreciating every moment I get to see interesting and exciting things for the first time, which is made even better if I'm with great people.

A dear friend was diagnosed with breast cancer a year before I had cervical cancer. We talked about the use of the word

"Survivor" in the recovery process. I told her I think the word and the timeframe for people to label themselves as a "Survivor" was invented to help people move on with their lives. To me it feels like an artificially derived label that psychologically puts an end date and start date in place. It falls into that routine of "managing expectations."

I'm sure it helps some people manage their expectations. For me, the kind of person who spends a lot of time in my head, and who is too practical for my own good at times, I believe no one is a "Survivor." Whether you have had cancer or haven't had it yet, the best chances you've got to survive anything are always 50-50 - A roll of the dice. There's a reason why Vegas calls it, Craps. The only way to increase the odds is to do what you can to stay out of the casino, out of harm's way, and focus on the half-filled glass with guarded optimism.

I believe there are Cancer Survivors and Cancer *Treatment* Survivors. I don't know if it's proper to capitalize both of those titles; but I did because they deserve the accolades of a proper noun. I'm a Cancer Treatment Survivor. Much of society tells me I can refer to myself as a Cancer Survivor once I hit the five-year mark. Unfortunately, many of the people I've met that had recurrence were beyond the five-year mark. The lady I mentioned early that I chatted with in the radiation waiting room had a recurrence after the five year mark, even though she had been proclaimed a "Survivor." My mom had breast cancer in 1978 at the age of fifty-two and is now an 87 year-old Cancer Survivor, but has severe Alzheimer's disease, which she will not survive. It seems one cannot get too over-confident about being a "Survivor." However, I suppose if a person must use labels to help him or her move forward, then that alone is enough of a utility to keep using them.

Cancer is the common denominator, but each person has unique facets to their life that make each cancer experience different for each person. All who have experienced cancer share the stages of diagnosis, surgery, treatment, recovery and rejuvenation. Some people check all the boxes, and sadly others don't. We relate to one another through the nuances of our individual stories. The shared experience allows the individual to have a sense of community, belonging, support, and belief that they can make it through the struggle. Others have gone before me, and therefore I had the courage to travel that same road.

One of my defense mechanisms during "the whole cancer thing" was to clinically observe myself as if I took one step back from the situation. After all, I was educated to observe human behavior and it was a big part of my previous job as a counselor. Why not turn my skills upon myself? Granted, the results of self-observation can be clouded with misinterpretations and wishful thinking. I know I'm being observed, which muddles the process and outcome. However, I can't stop doing it. Even better, I can write about it with the intent of helping others.

Once the two-year anniversary of surgery, chemo and radiation passed, I realized time seemed to be flying by faster than it used to. If I had to guess, I would say it was because I wasn't dreading my period every month. Dreading a monthly pain-in-the-ass female occurrence somehow slowed life down. Time has passed so quickly it still feels like 2010, which may be a by-product of my overall disconnection with life. Hitting the two-year cancer-free mark is a great feeling. Dr. T told me with cervical cancer, if there's going to be a recurrence it commonly happens within two years following treatment. While I want to believe what he says, I don't think I will ever feel 100 percent out-of-the-woods.

I believe if you have to face a new, additional and tough challenge while you're already feeling down, you tend to have an easier time managing the new situation. Basically, if I'm down, I can't go much further. I had cancer a second time in 2012. There was a spot on my arm that had bothered me for some time and I needed to get it checked. I figured I had already faced cancer head-on; so if this spot on my arm was going to be some form of carcinoma I could handle it.

My dermatologist took a biopsy and when his office called and told me it was cancer I actually had little to no reaction. Isn't that amazing? It could have been that I was still disconnected from most of my feelings subsequent to struggling through the torture of relentless nausea. I remember thinking, "Wow, I have no feeling about that."

I went back to the dermatologist and had a quarter size chunk of skin cancer removed from my arm. As the stink of burning flesh wafted into the air from cauterizing the edges of the wound, I realized a couple things. One: burning flesh is one of the sickest smells there is on the planet; and, Two: cancer had helped me develop some expanded levels of bravery.

The word "cancer" sends a lot of people to their knees. The true sign of bravery for me is to be afraid and do it anyway. Calling the dermatologist was scary; but having come through it the way that I did shows me my internal skill development is an ongoing process. Anyone who thinks they may have cancer should definitely have it checked out. You may end up showing yourself how brave you really are. However, I respect Mother Nature and never fully let go of the notion that utter terror can switch on in an instance.

Unfortunately, I had yet another scare when my mammogram came back with an issue in July of 2013. My mom had breast cancer so I was especially wary. The report mentioned that my breast tissue appeared to have a "summation" of tissue. For the better part of forty-eight hours I was feeling extremely, "forget-to-breathe" scared. I was most afraid of having to do anything that would involve nausea. I couldn't do that again. Now that I had first-hand knowledge of what was involved in the cancer journey, I was significantly more upset than when I didn't know what I didn't know. Ironically, being on the knowledgeable side helped me appreciate and fully understand the concept of ignorance is bliss.

My nerves were shot. I had enough distance away from my initial treatment to gain some confidence in my recovery - then POW! I thought I was back to square one. It felt similar to when you're learning to ski and you're doing pretty well. Then, you get a little cocky. The next thing you know you face-plant into the slope wondering what happened.

I went to my gynecologist's office and met with my favorite nurse practitioner, Michelle. She is the one who played a hunch and found my cancer in the first place. She counseled me on the issue and squelched my fear. Apparently I have what they call, "dense breasts," which I thought was a compliment at first. It wasn't. A repeat mammogram and an ultrasound determined that nothing was wrong.

In some ways I felt an emotional backslide, but eventually regrouped and moved forward. Truth be told, when and if the wolf comes knocking at my door, I will always run as fast as I can and hide my dense breasts from danger.

Trying to get my pause button unstuck has been a challenge. Through hard work and the help of Deborah, my counselor, I've learned many valuable things: I can't wait my turn for good things to happen. I have to make my turn. I have to be an active participant in those things that will move me physically, emotionally, spiritually and financially forward. I cannot participate in activities that hinder my belief in my ability to be successful in all areas of life.

Through the use of a therapeutic technique called EMDR (Eye Movement Desensitization and Reprocessing), Deborah has helped me shift and reprocess my thoughts about the life-damaging stress that was dished upon my plate during my journey. She has helped me solve some longstanding issues that hindered me from thriving in life. Her intelligence, care and specialty in helping cancer patients have made for a great working relationship. She was indispensable to my recovery and rejuvenation. Everyone should be so lucky, not just cancer patients. Without her help, I'm certain this book would not be a reality. It took two years for me to reach the point of starting to write this book. Each page that I write is an exercise in taking my life off of pause, which is so much better than pushing eject.

CH 10 -THE CAREGIVERS AND THEIR JOURNEY

If you're looking for a superhero for your next graphic novel, then strongly consider the likes of a caregiver who tends to the needs of a person dealing with cancer. The ones who do it with grace are the angels amongst us. If you are lucky like I was, they can singlehandedly enhance your healing process like nothing else. I made many discoveries in my personal journey; and in retrospect, want to share my thoughts.

Crisis renders most people difficult to deal with or at best to be inconsistent and short-tempered. Physical and/or emotional pain can be the most challenging thing to deal with in life. Frankly, the person who is unlucky enough to be by your side helping you push through and heal deserves respect of the highest accord. Unfortunately, many times that individual feels the brunt of your worst, which leaves you in a constant state of apology and/or guilt.

Many consider themselves either a fairly good caregiver or a horrible one. On the other hand, *wonderful* caregivers are usually so humble they shun any form of accolade for being a gift to others. Saying, "Thank you" over and over to your caregiver doesn't feel big enough when you are in an extremely compromising position.

Tireless, dutiful, focused, kind, loving, and generous are only a few of the qualities that a great caregiver brings to the relationship you forge from diagnosis to recovery and into rejuvenation. Often these people are not paid for their work while enduring the impact of cranky behaviors. It can become a formidable and sometimes horrendous situation that inevitably inflicts pain and may estrange families.

What doesn't readily occur to most is how to communicate their needs to the person who is trying to help. If a person is not able to articulate his/her needs, then the stage is set for a communication mishap. Unless you are aware of this necessity for communication prior to entering a caregiver-patient situation, it will likely go unaddressed. To make matters worse, there usually isn't someone to guide you through the course of action.

My suggestions: Each cancer patient should complete a questionnaire identifying as many of his or her needs and distinctive quirks destined to impact the caregiver–patient relationship. If not a questionnaire, then at least a discussion should take place between both. This would likely be the best gift you could give because this person will also be dealing with your plight. The caregiver will be experiencing their own arduous journey, which many times is even harder because they wish they could do more for you, but can't. I would venture to say the feelings of helplessness are equal to or even worse for the caregiver.

Undoubtedly, there will be a need for additional conversations throughout the progression of treatment because there will be a lot of first-time experiences for everyone involved. Advance preparation for the possibilities ahead is really helpful. Open communication will help manage challenges along the way.

This is a list of questions I developed, which arose from concerns that were obvious to me in the beginning of my situation and others that caught me by surprise as time passed:

1. Do you consider yourself a good or a bad patient?
2. Are you comfortable telling people when you are afraid?
3. What is your fear level regarding surgery in general?
4. How do you like to prepare yourself the day before the surgery?
5. Do you like to talk about the upcoming events or do you prefer to be quiet?
6. Do you consider your pain threshold high, medium, or low?
7. In what manner would you like people to ask you how you're feeling?
8. What type of environment helps you heal the best?
9. How do you deal with the unknown?
10. Do you consider yourself an anxious person?
11. How do you feel about being given unsolicited advice from others?
12. How do you usually deal with bad news?
13. What cheers you up like nothing else?
14. How willing are you to accept help of any kind?

15. If you are feeling nauseous, how do you want others to act around you?
16. Do you have any sensitivity to noises?
17. Do you have any sensitivity to smells?
18. What type of television shows do you not want to watch?
19. How comfortable are you with telling the doctor or nurses what you really need?
20. What is your biggest fear while in the hospital?
21. What is your biggest fear about chemotherapy?
22. What is your biggest fear about radiation?
23. What will be your sign when you want others to leave the room and let you rest?
24. How do you want to tell people that you're sick of all the attention and just want to be left alone for a while.
25. The last question is for the patient to ask the caregiver: What huge, elaborate, epic, incredible gift would you like to have once this job is complete?

In my particular situation, my partner, Barb, has a "love language" expressed through her fabulous cooking. When I was in the throes of relentless nausea, her favorite way to show she cared was rendered useless, even detrimental. The smell of most food made me sick. Even the taste of many foods was amplified to a point of disgust. I recall one afternoon when I looked out the window and saw a long orange electrical cord stretching about twenty feet with the end attached to a crock pot filled with the day's meal. How many people would do that for their loved one? Barb's efforts to help keep smells out of the house proved to me that love will find a way to shine through. As a matter of fact, her amazing banana bread was one of my go-to foods to help with nausea. For some reason the soft texture and mild taste soothed the savage upset, which was a welcome relief.

Today, some of the food that turned my stomach remains on that list. However, when the smell of freshly baked banana bread wafts through the air, I get excited. Although cancer makes you form some really negative associations, for me, banana bread will forever be associated with comfort. Yum! Keep those ripe bananas spoiling! They are the key to scrumptious delight.

I asked Barb what advice she would give to someone starting the caregiver trek for a cancer patient. She said one broad-brush comment, "I would tell them to get a support group around them." Can anyone hear the subtext in that statement like I can? Figure it out. Patients are high maintenance.

Most cancer transmigrations take a toll on everyone involved. I can't help but think a considerable amount of healing is needed to repair the harm. I would be considered lucky if it didn't create some permanent damage as well. As more good days, months, and years are connected, trust for a healthy future grows. Also, when the dust settled, I realized "the whole cancer thing" allowed me to see what unconditional love really looks like. Believe it or not, cancer gives gifts.

When the parties involved openly acknowledge the impact cancer can have on a relationship, the better the chances for successfully managing speed bumps along the way. The consequence is building a new vista to look out upon together. No one wants to be standing alone. Without love and understanding, relationships won't make it. It's like law school. A psychologist friend of mine who works at a law school told me that seventy-five percent of marriages or relationships fail by the time a law student finishes due to the impact of stress. I don't know the statistics, but I fear that many relationships are lost due to cancer. We worry about people leaving this life due to cancer. Unfortunately, a relationship can die from the cancer experience, which inflicts additional suffering to an already strained situation. Which is worse? You decide. All I'm saying is communicating your needs from the start and throughout the experience can likely save your relationships from certain death.

As they say in the teachings about active communication, "Seek first to understand then to be understood." When it comes to your cancer experience, understand that you and your relationships are going through an extremely demanding time. Clearly communicate your needs to help others understand you. It's not easy for anyone involved. Laying down clear boundaries could save you, and those you care about the most.

CH 11 - LET'S TALK ABOUT THE LEAD BALLOONS

Approximately one year before being diagnosed with cancer I ran into a friend in the lobby of the building that houses the chemotherapy infusion center. She was visiting a mutual friend who was doing a round of chemotherapy. I was in the building accompanying my mom who was getting her yearly mammogram. My mom is a 35-year survivor of breast cancer. Alzheimer's disease has taken the memory of cancer away, which is the *only* good thing about that horrible disease.

My friend and I were chatting and I introduced my mom to her. I threw out the fact that mom had survived the very cancer for which my other friend was being treated.

I turned to my mom and said, "Huh, mom?"

I looked at her and she began to tell my friend about surviving cancer and then shared something I hadn't ever heard her say. She shared how difficult it was for her to go back to work because everyone treated her differently. Friends she'd known for years were "stand-offish." This went on in varying degrees for the remainder of her years on the job. Her voice cracked and I saw tears well up in her eyes. My mom is a rock and to see her get emotional about her struggle some thirty-five years ago made me pause.

Let me put this in perspective. My mom had a mastectomy and was back to work in a couple of weeks. When she did chemotherapy, she never missed a day of work. Her chemotherapy consisted of drinking a chemo solution in orange juice every morning for five days, every six weeks for two years. Additionally, she managed a household with an extremely demanding husband and four kids who really didn't understand her plight. I cannot remember her ever wavering.

To shed light on how I really didn't understand: I remember telling my high school coach at the time that my mom was recovering from a *vasectomy*. When she slightly grinned and said, "You mean a *mastectomy*?" I corrected myself. Her grin didn't make sense to me until years later when I realized what I said.

For my mom, The Rock, to be brought to tears is a big thing. Her friends forever treated her differently after cancer. This may happen to any of us.

When we left the lobby that day, my mom and I talked about this in greater detail. She said the way her friends treated her was the hardest part of her cancer journey; harder than surgery, recovery and enduring two years of chemotherapy, which made her permanently nauseous at the slightest whiff of any lady's perfume. Every time she went to the doctor's office, the air was filled with an overpowering blend of perfumes that made my mom throw-up. Years later she still would get queasy each time she turned onto the street where the doctor's office was located. You think that's a trauma-based memory? Of course it is.

Cancer made my mom different; and each day a friend's silence or exclusion from participating in an event expanded the space between them. Luckily, my mom was very outgoing; and she made the best of it. Her closest friends restored her faith in friendships; but the only ones who *completely* understood were those who ended up with cancer themselves.

I have to remind myself at times that some people are really uncomfortable in situations that involve talking about feelings, experiencing feelings, and finding something to say during those situations. Working alongside my fellow counselors and with clients for seventeen years of my career definitely helped me build a level of ease with awkward moments. I'm actually quite comfortable with silence too. Go figure.

When a friend is seriously ill and dealing with life or death situations, some people cannot handle the upheaval, and will stay their distance. Without question, contemplating the thought of losing a friend to cancer is one of life's horrors. Some people are really good at showing up in those initial stages of "the whole cancer thing." Casseroles, cards and flowers are wonderful; but as time passes, attention subsides. Some people relish being removed from the limelight; others find it isolating and dismissive.

There was a distance I felt with some friends, and not with others. At times, I found myself purposely not talking about my recovery because I really didn't want to give the story any more airtime. A turning-point came when I needed to stop taking myself so seriously. Other times I just didn't want to share because it launched a lead balloon and created a dead spot in the conversation. Silence and stillness floated into the room as if we were suddenly playing a game of Freeze Tag.

I surmise that people back-off for all sorts of reasons. I remember in junior high and high school when all a girl had to do to get out of P.E. was mention her period. Teachers would squirm and back away from forcing the girl to do any kind of activity. Since I don't have my period to scare people off anymore, I decided mentioning cancer and my recovery would be my new tool for getting out of unwanted or boring conversations. You always need an out, right?

Observing others has always been part of who I am. Getting an under-graduate and graduate degree in the field of psychology was a natural fit. I am sincerely fascinated by human behavior. What we do to protect ourselves from others, our feelings and the world's pressure is incredibly complex. Nothing makes people squirm more than talking about cancer and death. It forces people to fumble with life's baggage. I write about it here because I want the reader to feel safe to face the awkwardness and hopefully reach a new level of understanding, strength and awareness.

Some people are concerned when they don't know what to say or do to make a situation better. There is a simple reality in all of this: sometimes you don't have to say anything at all. Silence is okay. Learn to be comfortable with it.

If you're looking for a "rule of thumb" about what to say, you should fault on the side of sticking with generally supportive statements such as: "I'm here for you in any way that I can be."; and "I will check in with you to see how you're doing."; and "My thoughts and prayers are with you."

Alternatively, if you are the person who is dealing with cancer, be open to those trusted individuals who want to hear your story. It allows your feelings to be *processed,* and will ultimately bring you peace.

I'm the type of person who is open to answer questions about my health. Sharing my experience might help others. Undoubtedly, it helps me re-establish balance in my life. The more information I can share with people, the more apt I am to process the feelings and emotions surrounding my experience. Telling my story is therapeutic – hence this book. Equally important to my balancing act is taking alone-time to recharge my batteries. The introverted-me wouldn't have it any other way.

If you're wondering what I said to the people who said ignorant or hurtful things during my journey, I calmly said, "Ouch, not helpful." It's all I could muster at the time. Hopefully, they will keep those kinds of comments to themselves in the future.

I can't expect people to be in tune with how they come across to others. However, every doctor, nurse practitioner, medical assistant and technician MUST be in tune with the needs of their patients. I can buffer myself from harm by allowing unwanted comments to bounce off; and grant myself the freedom to imagine sending a few expletives their way if I feel the need.

One instance in particular deserves further discussion. During my pre-op diagnostics, it was discovered that I had a borderline dilation in my aorta. Although it was determined not to be a health risk, it was suggested that I have this issue monitored. About seven months post-chemo and radiation, I scheduled and attended an appointment to have a body scan that included six or seven types of tests. A cardiac ultrasound was included, as was screening for peripheral artery disease, a carotid arteria ultrasound, and a couple of others. The price was only $179, which was hundreds of dollars cheaper than just the co-pays if I were to go through my insurance. The tests were administered in these really cool, ultra-equipped medical mobiles. I arrived on time for my appointment and took a seat inside the make-shift medical facility. I'm always friendly at medical appointments, which sometimes backfires. When I happily greeted the technician who would be performing the diagnostic tests, she smiled and was friendly in return. She walked me back to the area, reached for the sliding accordion door, turned and looked at me, smiled a big smile and said, "Welcome to the *death* chamber."

Also, it happened to be the Monday after Superbowl and she and the other technician were making light of having clogged arteries sustained by eating crappy food at a party the day before. These were such incredibly insensitive things to say that I looked around to see if I was being punked, was the victim of a *Candid Camera*-reboot TV show, or an unwitting participate on *Dateline NBC's "What would you do?"* I was speechless. Fortunately, I could laugh about the absurdity of the event later because I was still pretty much detached from my feelings.

How could the mobile technician know that I was only seven months out from a life-or-death predicament? She couldn't. The point is: she should **not** be saying such things to anyone at any time. There should be a zero-tolerance policy. I called the company's customer service department once I got home and calmly advised them what happened. I told them I didn't expect too much to happen as a result; but I had to be heard.

Before a word is uttered, people need to think through all the possible consequences of what they say to someone who is going through cancer surgery and treatment. When in doubt, silence is probably your best bet if you think something harmful will come out of your mouth due to your own awkwardness. Just breathe and be there for the person. Keep it simple. We, the people experiencing the cancer, can feel awkward about your awkwardness. If everyone just calms down it can solve most any challenge.

The cancer experience is isolating. It made me feel like climbing into a cave to hide from life. When the time was right, I pulled myself out of that cave and stepped into the light again. Friendships were the handrails that made the ascent possible. In turn, my friends remembered that with time came an opportunity to welcome me back. We, the cancer "peeps," struggle with that concept every day. To have a friend sidle up next to me and help me feel part of life again is one of the greatest gifts to give - that, and really tasty desserts.

The palpable disconnect people might feel can't be generating entirely from an outside source. It is reasonable to think the distance could be emanating from inside the mind, body, and soul of the person dealing with cancer. Who knows? What I do know is that it is real; and I wanted to talk about it in this book because it's part of the whole cancer experience. There is a silent sort of bias that happens that feels like you've been excluded or are being treated with kid gloves. Not in a weepy kind of "I'm a victim" way. That's what it felt like to me. It was not a good feeling, but one that could be managed by extending myself back into a world that has so much to offer.

My sense of safety shifted during "the whole cancer thing"; and keeping a distance felt safe to me. The danger comes when a healthy distance becomes prolonged isolation. I made a concerted effort to balance the frequency and intensity of social interactions in a way that did not overwhelm me.

It was not about forcing myself back into society, but rather making healthy social interactions part of a balanced life. The fun part is being really choosy about with whom you spend time. I had cancer, and I found myself shuffling, categorizing and prioritizing relationships in a way that allowed me to only spend quality time with quality people for quality reasons.

If you live long enough, your life will be touched by cancer in some way. If it touches you, sometimes others may not know what to do for you, with you, or know how to behave around you. That's okay.

When my mom had cancer in 1978 there were no programs available to talk about any of the fallout that happens during the journey. Today there are wonderful programs and therapists available to those in need.

I wrote this book to tell my story, but to also tell my mom's story so people will realize the importance of staying connected with those experiencing cancer. It's also essential to know that we definitely don't want this connection out of pity. Welcoming those folks back into life will be the kindest thing you may ever do. Don't forget to bring a yummy dessert.

One last thing:

Dear Friends,

You are in my life for a reason. Sharing my experience with you makes us closer; and knowing you are there for me in whatever way you can brings me great healing. I will be here for you in turn if cancer or any other challenge comes knocking on your door. I will be sensitive to your needs and support you in any way I can. I will check in on you to ensure that you know I care. I will call first before showing up with casserole in hand; and I promise never to minimize your struggles. If you want to be alone, I will respect your wishes. I will advocate for you and kindly, or not, pounce on anyone I have to in order to address your needs. I am here with you, always.

Much love,

Anne

"Live Life To Write About It." – Anne Kruse

CH 12 - I'LL TAKE YOU THROUGH THE FOLLOW-UP

My follow-up plan originally consisted of appointments with my gynecological oncologist, chemotherapy oncologist, and radiation oncologist. During the first couple of months after surgery and treatment, I had weekly visits. The remainder of the first two years I had appointments every ninety days. Collectively, the follow-up appointments consisted of blood work, scans, and gynecological exams every three months. I know some people who only have gynecological exams once every three to five years. Aren't you lucky? For the men reading this book, close your eyes and imagine a prostate exam or other invasive cavity search happening every ninety days. Sound like fun?

Luckily for me, the facility where my gynecological oncologist resides is a fantastic environment and the staff is top-notch. I was actually the first person to have surgery through their newly established center/department within a well-established hospital system. The lobby always has really good coffee, cookies, and a big TV that plays ocean scenes on a loop. I feel safe there and that makes it easier. I'm committed to the protocol for follow-up. Small complaints aside, I'm fortunate and happy to be receiving the crucial care I need.

At the two-year mark my gynecological oncologist, Dr. T, extended the time between my appointments to once every six months, as did my chemo oncologist, Dr. P. I stopped seeing my radiological oncologist after approximately three months because it just seemed like a redundancy that could be eliminated. It wasn't hard to get used to this since the awful nurse, Agnes, was in that office (see Chapter 7). Never seeing that woman again would be fabulous. Unfortunately, I have to pass by her office on my way to the chemo oncologist. She triggers something really agitating inside of me: fight-or-flight response in full regalia. Keeping my own leash held tight at this point seems to manage my urge to get arrested.

There is a psychological pattern that I've fallen into during follow-up. I set the appointment and then put it out of my mind until one week before. The night before my obligatory visit I tell myself that I've just got to get to the office, and by noon the next day it will all be over. I practice my breathing exercises during my stay and try to smile as much as possible, even if I fake it until I make it. I'm friendly to all the staff and they are in return. All staff members at Dr. T's office are exceptional in their field. The "powers that be" hired the cream of the crop when the hospital decided to start this special program.

A few miles away at my chemo oncologist, Dr. P's office, the staff is quite opposite in character. The first thing I notice and feel is the complete lack of smiling people behind the desk and in the back office. It's awful. You can't get a smile out of any of them. Believe me, I try. If I put my career counselor hat on, I would venture to say they really don't like their jobs and should find another line of work. It's time to update some resumes. I believe they have forgotten that a big part of their duty is to HELP people who have cancer, are recovering from cancer, and are probably having a much worse day than they are. I've already voiced my opinion through a customer care questionnaire, but have not seen any improvement - perhaps next time, or *perhaps* never. I've done my part and will continue to be gracious when I visit them in hopes of one day getting at least a slight grin in return.

This office fills with people in various stages of their journey. I see people who are there for their first appointment with family members coming in one-by-one as each exclaims their struggle to find parking. There are those who walk in, get wheeled in, or use their walkers and canes. There are people who look near death and people who exude lively energy. Seeing all those folks in the waiting room was very difficult for me in the beginning. It continues to pull at my heart strings. I try to focus on myself and breathe my way through the tough spots and be friendly to everyone.

The simplest things like making an appointment can be overwhelming. I'm writing about this because that is what I had to do today. I called the office of my gynecological oncologist, Dr. T, to make an appointment. The last time I was in I was told to call in September to set an October appointment. Here's how the call went:

VICTORIA AT THE OFFICE:

Hello, Cancer Prevention and Treatment Center, this is Victoria. How may I help you?

ME:

Hello Victoria, this is Anne Kruse. How are you?

VICTORIA:

Just fine Anne. How are you?

ME:

I'm well. I was told to give a call in September to make an appointment for October.

VICTORIA:

Okay. Is this a three month follow-up?

ME:

No, it's a six month follow-up.

VICTORIA:

Oh that's great! Let's see what Dr. T has open. He's got October, 7th, 21st and the 28th. He's going to be out on the 14th.

ME:

Let's do the 21st.

VICTORIA:

How's 10:00 a.m.?

ME:

That will work.

VICTORIA:

Okay, we'll see you then, Anne.

ME:

Thank you.

...And scene.

I know that sounds as easy as making a hair appointment; but other than the potential for a bad haircut there are no life-or-death thoughts you have to deal with when calling your hair stylist. Each time I have to make an appointment I'm forced to open myself up to the possibility that there will be a recurrence; and I will know about it in less than a month. I purposely make it a month ahead to mentally prepare for the appointment. For the next 30 days I will be vacillating between waves of terror sprinkled with denial. Yes, a little bit of denial helps soften the edges. The art of effectively disconnecting from your feelings is also important to have at-the-ready in your hip pocket.

It is so interesting to notice things happening within me. For most of my adult life I've tried to practice connecting mind with body and spirit. During these thirty day progressively knuckle-whitening experiences, I turn up the efforts to disconnect my mind from my body. Yes, of course it's a defense mechanism.

As a writer, I have honed my ability to wait for things to happen and people to respond. This requires me to stunt my feelings to the point of barely caring about anything. I tell myself that waiting for appointments and results are not as hard as waiting to hear back from someone about a writing project I've worked on for years. Isn't that sad? The writer's life can be more difficult than managing cancer and what comes your way. Sometimes I slow time down. I just nestle into a moment and think to myself, "Right here in this moment, I don't have cancer and I feel great. I won't have to worry about anything until I absolutely have to worry about it." This simple thought is a perfect example of staying in the present moment. It's a nice place to visit.

The day before my appointment I seem to get increasingly quiet. It's like I'm sneaking around trying to hide from Mother Nature should she decide to tap me on the shoulder and ask me to leave. Also, I notice that my breathing gets shallow and my appetite lessens. Remembering to breathe becomes a requirement because I catch myself thinking my way into paralysis about the "what ifs" that could be on the horizon. My arms get heavy. I feel unsettled. I'm more sensitive to noises than usual. I think this is directly tied to my fight-or-flight response, which takes a thrashing during this time.

The morning of the appointment I limit my caffeine intake to keep myself calm. I try to eat a decent breakfast because I don't want to get lightheaded, which I have done at other appointments.

It is absolutely essential to make sure I have enough time to avoid any type of rush to my doctor visit, or even worse, be late. By the time I'm behind the wheel I'm focused on the task at hand: getting my appointment over and returning home. I've noticed plenty of spikes in the frequency of my road rage while traveling to my rendezvous point. It feels like people are in my way and I've got to get this arduous duty completed as soon as possible. I let them know by yelling at them with my *windows closed*. It's super-effective.

The Center has valet parking and I happily take advantage of it to avoid dealing with a crowded multi-level parking structure. The valets are always so helpful and considerate. They know they are the first "greeters" people encounter before entering the building. They set the tone for a doctor visit. Of course, I'd rather be going to a nice restaurant or somewhere that warrants special parking. It's worth the $8.00 to hasten the process, which brings me closer to it being over.

The drop-off area is the first place you are reminded that people dealing with cancer are all around. The hardest ones for me to see are the frail, elderly folks and little toddlers. On numerous visits I saw a three-year-old boy who had to wear a helmet to protect the surgical site of an operation he had on his skull. His mom carried him like a mom does, and I thought about how difficult it must be for her. Of course I worried about the boy, but I worried more about her because I wondered if she had someone caring about her. She was in crisis mode, so I get it. The point is I KEPT seeing her and her boy; and that meant that he was still here, with his family, living life. Even if I don't see her at my next appointment, I know that it doesn't necessarily mean that the little boy died. I tell myself he just happened to finish with his treatment and he's getting better. Telling made-up stories is one way to manage the reality of the situation. I do enjoy storytelling.

Once inside The Center I stop at the registration desk to verify my insurance. I use this opportunity to measure my recovery.

The rule at the facility requires you to register once each month during your treatment. Early on there was a time when I had multiple appointments in a month and could just walk straight into my doctor's office without stopping at the registration desk. Now, since I'm scheduled for follow-up appointments every six months, I have to register each time. It's an inconvenience I relish. Sometimes there's no line and that makes it that much sweeter.

I know I mentioned before that my doctor's waiting room has to be one of the best waiting rooms ever designed (peaceful ocean scenes on TV, coffee and cookies). Obviously they paid close attention to every detail. The ambience and food diversions are appreciated. I practice a calming technique called, "tapping" that allows me to manage the moment. Deep breaths are helpful and cell phone distractions are too; but the cell signal isn't very good, which is probably related to the heavy-duty medical machinery zapping away in the building.

An office/medical assistant comes out into the lobby and calls me in to begin the routine. I truly appreciate each member of the permanent staff. Shannon is great. She weighs me, takes vitals and ensures I've got all that I need. She will always hold a special place in my journey. She is the one who helped me celebrate my ability to pee when the catheter was removed. She also was instrumental in finding and ordering smaller speculums for the clinic, which makes me very happy. For the record, one size does not fit all. Apparently, others have benefitted from my tenacity to get more comfortable equipment. I'm glad I spoke up.

Dr. T always has an underling doctor participating in a three-month fellowship join him during the visit. In addition to Dr. T, I've had many different doctors perform the pap and pelvic exams. Dr. T's technique is considerably better. It's uncomfortable, but he really is very mindful, and confident. As far as the other doctors, plain and simple, the female doctors are the best - probably because they know what it feels like. The world would benefit from them helping their male counterparts polish their technique. Some of the male doctors I simply did not trust, and asked in a kind way if Dr. T could perform the exam.

To my shock, at my last appointment, the doctor who walked into the exam room was none other than, Dr. Gruff. If you recall, he was the doctor I met the morning of my surgery who said some things that pissed me off. He helped Dr. T in surgery. I believe he's responsible for the heinous, crooked and gathered, eleven-inch scar cascading down the length of my abdomen. Note to anyone out there: make sure you ask the doctor if they took sewing in junior high school; because lack of that skill could instigate a scar like mine. Unfortunately, the great seamstresses amongst the nation's doctor-crew become plastic surgeons. I was advised by Colleen, the Nurse Navigator to ask for the plastic surgeon to be part of my surgical team. I failed to do that for no other reason than I was so overwhelmed by everything before surgery and forgot to ask. Insurance won't cover it now.

Well, I decided to move forward with the exam and allow Dr. Gruff to perform it. Unfortunately, I will never describe him as someone with finesse. In fact, it's way more painful than it should be. I assumed every doctor specializing in the area of gynecological oncology was an expert in female anatomy. Next time, if he's the doctor on duty, I will ask to have Dr. T perform the exam. Life's too short to allow Gruff in your nether regions.

I am actually writing this portion of the book one week after my six month follow-up visit with Dr. T. On the day of the appointment I got a call telling me Dr. T was called into surgery and he wouldn't be in the office until 10:00 a.m. My appointment was scheduled for 10:00 and there were six patients ahead of me on the schedule. They were looking for people to reschedule. I had put myself through such a process of mental preparedness there was no way I was going to change and have to start over. Instead, I went in two hours late and it all worked out.

My nurse navigator, Colleen, whom I adore, came into the lobby before my appointment to say hello. She pulled me aside to tell me that a particular resident who was working in a fellowship under Dr. T was back in the clinic due to a rotation schedule. We will call him, Dr. Flunk. He would have received a failing grade for his performance in initial patient interaction at my prior visit during the first year of follow-up. For what it's worth, there was a point in my life when I had two roommates who were studying to be doctors. They would practice their clinical skills (non-invasive) on me in preparation for tests. I'm well-versed in the protocol, which makes me painfully aware of when a doctor's skills are less than acceptable and not in line with what they were trained to perform.

The previous appointment with Dr. Flunk started with him entering the exam room displaying a body posture and attitude that could best be described as lackadaisical. Based on body language alone, it seemed he was just stopping by to give me a flu shot. This guy is dealing with patients at various stages of the cancer journey! First he pronounced my name wrong, which happens. Then, he got my surgery date wrong. Next, he thought I was going to have chemo when I had already finished, which made me want to barf.

After these not-so-charming botch-ups he said, "Boy, I bet you're saying this guy doesn't know what he's doing."

I said, "You are correct."

He was the only one chuckling. Come on! At least try to read something about a patient before coming in the room! My two doctor friends would have first kicked his ass, then laughed him out of the clinic.

I clearly understand the need to be flexible with all fellowship doctor/interns coming in and out of the clinic every three months. Based on necessity, I devised a little three-prong evaluation for any doctor with whom I come in contact. If they got three pieces of information about me wrong, then I needed to say something. My trust of anyone and everyone had been damaged through the cancer process. A plan of action helped me watch out for myself as I tried to build trust in others.

At minimum I expect doctors to scan my chart before talking to me, for obvious reasons. When I'm struggling through a "trust-no-one" phase, I can tell you that someone like Dr. Flunk did nothing to establish trust or even anything remotely akin to a patient-doctor relationship. I trust my dry cleaner more than Dr. Flunk; and my dry cleaner has lost a few favorite articles of my clothing. Basically, I stopped any further discussion and calmly told him that I would wait to see Dr. T rather than continue our interaction. A medical appointment is all about the patient! All efforts and actions need to be focused, caring and emotionally healing. Dr. Flunk did not demonstrate any level of understanding for that universal truth.

I wrote an email to Colleen, the Nurse Navigator, to make her aware of what happened. She told me at our initial meeting that her role and function in the clinic is to make sure everyone is doing their job. During my visit, I knew I was doing my job by being congenial, attentive and cooperative. Dr. Flunk was not doing his. Frankly, if my initial interaction with him was his job interview, I would have cut it short at five minutes and moved on to the next applicant.

The Center has done an excellent job of staffing each position with great people who aspire to help patients suffering intense and dire circumstances. They remain positive and realize the task at hand: helping people stare cancer in the eye and try to find a way to eliminate it for good. It is clear that the staff aspires to be outstanding. Dr. Flunk did not demonstrate any level of aspiration in my opinion. I find it hard to believe that he would have acted the same way in front of Dr. T knowing he was a participant in his fellowship. Dr. T couldn't be more opposite in his demeanor and bedside manner. He has a superior ability for talking about the harsh realities of cancer. It is a true gift.

Back to my recent visit. Colleen told me that Dr. Flunk was there and asked me if I preferred not to see him because of the bad experience I had. The fact that she remembered, almost a year prior, really told me she had my back. These are the kinds of behaviors that help a patient rebuild trust, which is priceless. And yes, of course I said, "No thank you" to the prospect of seeing Dr. Flunk again.

We went through the routine of the exam: Pap smear and pelvic exam. Dr. T said everything looked good and the lab results would be available in about a week or so. Even though we make small talk, it's usually quite meaningful. This visit he told me that he always remembers the people involved rather than the actual surgery. He told me that he always remembers what a great advocate Barb was for me and how kind she was. Then, he said something that scared the crap out of me. He also remembered that before the surgery they weren't sure if they were going to be able to remove all of the cancer and may have had to close me back up. This wasn't new information, but now it seemed I misunderstood something Dr. Gruff told me on the day of my surgery.

About a week before surgery I met with Dr. Dainty Hands, as previously described in an earlier chapter, and she went down her checklist of things to discuss. One of the usual things that a patient is told prior to a surgery is that there is always the possibility that they would get in and it might be worse than anticipated. They might have to close you back up. I figured this was routine. All diagnostics at that juncture were pointing to a surgery that would go as planned.

The morning of the surgery as I'm sitting in pre-op in my gown, shower cap, and slightly sedated into a lull, Dr. Gruff came to visit me, who I had not met. He introduced himself and said he was working in a fellowship with Dr. T and would be assisting in the surgery. He went on to tell me that there was a possibility that they would get in there and might not be able to do the surgery to remove all the cancer. I thought he was going through the same routine that I had already heard from Dr. Dainty Hands, when in fact this apparently was NEW information that was conveyed from Dr. T and told to me. I told him, "Yes, I'm aware of that. I was told that in my pre-op appointment. Why are you telling me that now? I'm nervous enough." He just nodded.

The clarity of this information came into focus during my visit last week, two years and nine months after surgery. It wasn't routine information. It was NEW information that shed light where I really didn't need it to be shone. Strangely, I, who asks questions about things like that didn't want to know anything more from Dr. T as he stood in front of me. I believe I responded to him by simply saying, "Yep."

We finished up the exam and Dr. T advised that recurrence usually happens within the first two years after surgery; so things are looking good. I am three months away from my three year anniversary of my surgery and will continue on an every-six-month schedule for another year and a half. Each visit is a milestone and I celebrate it with the staff. They appreciate success stories and you can really see it in their faces. Their eyes have seen the horrors of what cancer can do; and I know their celebrations with me are genuine. They have earned my trust and continue to impress me each time I visit.

Dare I say I had fun at my cancer follow-up visit? I wished everyone a happy holiday season and they did me the same. I had a final chat with Victoria at the front desk and told her that I was writing this book, which she said she would love to read. Victoria, if you're reading this – I actually did it!

As a matter of routine, I usually hit the produce market on the way home from a visit to pick up some healthy, fresh food. It always feels like a solid act of good health, which helps celebrate getting the visit out of the way. Later, the visit's completion was celebrated with butternut squash gnocchi and a trip to the movies. Mission accomplished.

Navigating through the follow-up period feels a bit like I'm living in six-month intervals as if they are an entire lifetime; but I'm starting to stitch together these segments to make it seem more like one continuous stream. I'm not completely over the mental hiccups that follow-up visits create in my life, but I'm healing and getting better with each one. It will always be a part of life that has to be managed. Finding the right tools and strategies to do that, is part of the journey. When you feel well-equipped you simply feel better, which allows you to plug into the process and move forward.

There may be additional hiccups during the follow-up period that are not anticipated, which will likely add turmoil to a person's life. It is bound to happen. For example, in April of 2014 my medical insurance got cancelled. Luckily for me, The Affordable Care Act had been enacted and I was able to secure a policy. Due to a tax technicality I was not eligible for any discounts. However, I was able to secure an individual policy that allows me to continue treatment with my doctors. It didn't seem very wise to secure a minimal catastrophic-only policy. I decided on a policy that covers eighty percent of most services and has no deductible. Obviously, I had to choose a policy that covered the worst case scenario. The fee for such a thing at this point is $558.00 per month, which just increased from my initial rate eight months ago of $503.00 per month. How am I able to pay such a high rate? I'm not, and cringe each month my debt gets higher and higher. Does the phrase, "Stuck between a rock and a hard place," come to mind?

When all is said and done, I know I need insurance because cancer may return. I'm lucky I can get a policy even though I've had cancer. The Affordable Care Act made it illegal to deny medical coverage due to preexisting conditions. Without The Act I definitely would have been denied coverage. Approximately seven years ago I applied for an individual policy with Kaiser and they turned me down just because I took a minimal dose of thyroid medication for a sluggish thyroid. What hope would I have had to get one with cancer on my record? Answer: none.

A recent visit to my gynecologist's office for well-woman care tells me things are looking up. When I found out I had cancer I got the best customer service possible, which is a great thing if your life needs saving. On the flip side of that I remember looking forward to a time when I would return to getting less than great customer service because that was an indication I was no longer high on the totem pole.

The customer service experience I had recently in the lobby while waiting to see Michelle, my life-saving Nurse Practitioner, was a sure sign of good things to come. I arrived on time for my 9:00 a.m. appointment and ended up being ignored and brushed aside. I waited an hour and a half before getting to see Michelle.

If getting bad customer service at my doctor's office means I'm not on the top of the totem pole and out-of-danger, then this brings me solace. All kidding aside, a cancer patient does not want to feel minimized or pushed to the side or forgotten. I've been fighting for my life; and I'm probably a bit feistier when provoked. It's funny what true life or death experiences will do to a woman's assertiveness. More importantly, everyone deserves to receive reasonable customer service; and I will do what I must to never be ignored. I can thank cancer for that. So, great news: I'm officially getting less than great customer service. Recovery is well on its way!

"Live Life To Write About It." – Anne Kruse

CH 13 - NAUSEA NEEDS ITS OWN CHAPTER

I have met people who pride themselves on having a "no-barf" record. My sister, Lisa, at one point had not barfed in over twelve years. When her record was broken a few flu seasons ago, she was angry her achievement whooshed away with a flush of the toilet. She said she did everything she could not to barf in hopes of keeping her record alive. The facts are plain and simple: most people do not like to barf, and they will conjure up whatever mind-game possible to resist the urge.

I didn't throw-up much as a child. I do remember a few occasions waking up and tossing my cookies in bed. Another time I hurled in the doorway of a large department store. Admittedly, there were a few bouts with the stomach flu that took me to my knees. As an adult, most of my regurgitation has been attributed to a food-related upset, or my physical intolerance to alcohol.

In 2007 when I cared for my dog, Takota, during his fatal journey with a rare lymphoma, I felt nauseous a lot. Perhaps it was the helpless feeling brought about by his struggle. All I know is that since then my nausea trigger gets easily pulled.

In the 1990's when I got my wisdom teeth removed I had no problem with nausea after coming out of general anesthesia. However, by the time I had throat surgery in 2008 to remove half of my thyroid gland and a tangerine size nodule, I was nauseous and hurling on a regular basis following anesthesia. Oh yes, this happens even after receiving that magic shot the anesthesiologist gives you to help you not barf!

After throat surgery not only did I get sick from the anesthesia, I found out the hard way I was allergic to morphine. As I watched the nurse inject my IV with a dose of morphine, a swell of nausea hit me like a tsunami. I immediately had to grab a bucket and let it fly. For the next five hours I was miserable and had an epic headache. The doctor finally contacted the nurse's station and wrote an Rx for Tylenol and codeine, which to this day is the only heavy pain med that doesn't make me sick. Most heavy-duty pain medications are just too much for my system to handle. There is something ironically cruel when pain medication causes you new and different pain. I'm sticking with over-the-counter ibuprofen as my "go-to" pain reliever whenever possible.

I went into chemotherapy and radiation with somewhat of an open mind. I was told that "some people" don't even get nauseous. A girl can only hope to be on the positive side of that folk tale. I was feeling really good going into the process. Surgery was almost six weeks behind me. I was eating well, healing well and felt truly sound. Dare I say I was feeling strong? How hard could it be?

Day one of chemotherapy the nausea started and six agonizing weeks later it stopped. It was the closest thing to being in prison that I have ever felt. Who knows? I've never been to prison so it may be worse. I quickly found out that I wasn't one of the lucky "some people" noted above. Are there really living, breathing human beings who don't get nauseous with chemo and radiation? It's probably another thing the doctors tell you to shoot you with a positive-placebo in hopes you'll be influenced simply by their words. Persuasion for me is a little tougher to come by. I want to believe, but it just doesn't happen.

Food smells, dog breath, soaps, candles, you name it and it made me feel like I was going to get sick. It really made me wonder about why our bodies have that mechanism. On an evolutionary level, bad smells are supposed to warn us about dangerous foods and environmental cautions. What could it mean when most everything with a smell sets off a danger signal so profound that you want to get as far away, and as fast as possible?

I spent most of my "sick as a dog" sentence curled up on the couch with my eyes shut. I would watch TV but the light from it hurt my eyes. I experienced a sensation that felt like items in the room were shooting and poking into my right eye; so I would close it most of the time. A fever gives me the same feeling. The doctor couldn't explain why this was happening, other than to say it was a side effect. All I know is that it was happening. As a matter of fact, I just recently stopped shutting my right eye when I watch TV. Although I still suffer some pain and sensitivity in my right eye, shutting it became a habit, which two-plus years later I'm attempting to break.

When I was relentlessly nauseous, I realized how many food commercials are on television; and was astonished at how many food shows I watched. The mute button on the remote became my friend. My food shows had to go on hiatus while I was undergoing treatment. I'm certain their ratings went down.

Some memories from that time come rushing back without warning. I remember a commercial about a hotel in Las Vegas with annoying, scratchy, world-beat music that played over and over. A year or so later the commercial started playing again and I immediately turned it off as fast as I could. That trauma-memory is still inside me and I want none of it. I didn't even like Vegas in the first place.

It surprises even me to know that I don't suffer from writer's block. In fact, it's the opposite. I have too many ideas to write about. However, this chapter about nausea did cause me to pause. In order to put myself into a place where I can write about my experience I muster up the feelings that I was feeling during that time. These are feelings I don't want to feel, let alone hunt down and relive just so I can write about them. However, my willingness to tangle with dry heaves is a no-brainer if I stand a chance of helping another person who is feeling the same way. I'm not the only one that has felt this kind of debilitation. Somehow when you read about other people's struggle and know that it finally subsides, you can tie a knot in that rope and hold on.

The first day of chemotherapy I was set up with an arsenal of anti-nausea medications. They were put in a designated area at my house with a schedule listing all the times I was supposed to take a dose. I was counseled repeatedly about staying on schedule with the drugs because if the hurling got out of control it would be hard to get back under control. Mine was never under control. I shouldn't say, never. The only time it was under control was when I was getting the drug in an IV. Taking the pill form of medication just wasn't being assimilated by my body. The conclusion: Nothing other than IV drugs worked very well.

While sitting in the chemo chair for eight hours, I finally found relief from crashing waves of queasiness. I had poisonous chemicals being pumped into my veins, but surprisingly I was weathering the storm. Go figure. Within an hour or two after completing the chemo treatment, the curse was back. That feeling would creep up and all I wanted to do was cry. It was the worst, most uncomfortable sense of doom.

At night I was told to take Benadryl to help with my restlessness, a side-effect of the anti-nausea medication. The feeling is best described as being compelled to keep my legs moving because it would help manage the buzzing, nervous, anxious sensitivities I was having. That doesn't make any logical sense, but it didn't stop me from moving my legs. You pull out whatever works if you have to.

The last thing I would do before trying to go to sleep was take a bite of banana bread. It was important that my stomach was not empty; and the banana bread was just the right texture and density to make that happen. It brought me great comfort then and still does today. I had some this morning as a matter of fact. Each yummy bite might remind me of chemo and radiation, but banana bread was a huge bright spot in all the darkness.

Trying to eat the proper amount of food during the day was difficult. I was force-feeding myself. There wasn't a time when I ever felt hungry. It's as if food had to be put on my schedule so I would make sure to eat. Previously when starving my way through a fad diet or other mode for healthy weight loss, I would have paid big bucks to have this same feeling. Good timing has never been my friend. In fact, cancer completely stole my thunder when my sister and I lost close to twenty pounds each the summer before I was diagnosed. When I saw people I hadn't seen in a while they thought I had lost weight because of the cancer instead of acknowledging my huge summertime accomplishment. Granted I did lose an additional five-to-seven pounds over the course of treatment, but can a girl catch a break?

Food wasn't the only thing I had to force into my body. Remember that I had to force myself to drink thirty-two ounces of water two hours before my radiation appointment and hold it until the radiation treatment was complete? I'm sure everyone has had to hold their pee at some point in their life; but doing it every day when you're already nauseous, weak, beaten down and exhausted makes it unbearable. To make matters worse, I usually had to take a shower before going to radiation. When the warm water hit, it took all I could muster to not be like a sleepy "tween" girl at a slumber party whose hand has been placed in a warm bowl of water. I see people competing on TV shows doing all sorts of crazy things. Try holding your pee for three hours and see who doesn't wet their pants. I won't be auditioning for that show any time soon.

My focus during radiation was to get into the treatment room, up on the table, have the two-minute treatment, then run straight to the bathroom to empty my bladder. Every time I made it to the toilet it took a little coaxing to let my bladder finally relax and let it all go. Relief was one of the most positive emotions experienced during my treatment. It's still one of my favorites.

If I'm going to talk about nausea then I've got to talk about medical marijuana. From a pure observer's point of view I was amazed by quite a few things. First of all, I live in California; and while I was in treatment there were many medical marijuana dispensaries in operation close to my home. They were legal in California, but the Federal Law prohibited them. This is one of those odd predicaments when the laws haven't caught up with social change. Bottom line: if you wanted to seek help with nausea via medicinal marijuana you were going to be violating a Federal Law, and California was happy to help me do it.

I suppose I should start this story by admitting that I was never a big pot smoker. The sensation it gave me was not anything I would classify as, "enjoyable." My friends *enjoyed* laughing at me especially when I thought everyone was trying to take pictures of me and show them to my parents. Remember, this was way before everyone carried a phone with a camera. I was jealous that I never felt the same relaxation my friends did after smoking pot. I wish I had. It made me paranoid and hungry for off-beat creative food (peanut butter, cheese whiz and jelly bean sandwiches). I worried about forgetting who I was and wandering off, but was hesitant to being put on a leash. There is no way anyone would enjoy feeling what I felt. No way. I take that back. The creative "food projects" where astonishingly good; and nowadays would *easily* be worthy of a phone-photo to share with my social media friends.

This was more than thirty years ago. Everyone I know who still smokes pot told me that the cultivation of marijuana has improved; and it is possible to get marijuana that helps with specific maladies. The pot industry went on without me for thirty-plus years so I was out-of-the-loop. However, the nausea I was experiencing pulled me back into the loop out of desperation.

My prescribed medication had very little impact. Although the drug I received in my IV on the day of chemo worked, there was a limit on how many treatments I could have. Regrettably, the one thing that worked was limited by my insurance company, which felt like a crime against humanity.

I decided to ask people in the chemo and radiation centers if they knew anything about how to get medicinal marijuana. Based on the stunned look on everyone's face, you would have thought I was asking where I could score an eight ball of cocaine or get a good price on a prostitute. It was absolutely amazing. Perhaps they were afraid of legal ramifications. Some people I asked were cool about it but honestly didn't know; and they even asked me to tell them once I found out. Yes, I was going to become an informant. I was willing to walk that slippery slope if it meant I could get a break from the nausea.

My view about marijuana usage is similar to any other drug or substance that alters your reality: there is a utility to all of them. As long as the use of such things does not contribute to harming an innocent bystander, or interfere with the health of a relationship, they can be used in moderation.

Since no one I spoke with knew anything about where or how to get medicinal marijuana, I decided to do some research. If anything, it was going to be interesting to discover more about this thing that was baffling all the medical workers. I now had a purpose.

When I told my sister, Kathi, about their reactions, she sprang into action. She too was fascinated that no one in the medical community knew where or how to score some weed. Based on steadfast internet perusing, we found a conveniently located dispensary. We were informed that a patient must get a "recommendation" from a doctor; and then that "recommendation" would allow me to purchase as much marijuana as I needed. Sounds easy, right? It was one of those moments in life when I thought if someone told me thirty years ago it was going to be this way in the future, I would have concluded it was a hallucination. My friends would have hoped it was true, but they wouldn't have believed it either.

I talked to my oncologist and told him about needing a "recommendation." He had not heard about this, but was willing to write on a prescription pad the following: "Patient in chemotherapy. Patient may benefit from medicinal marijuana." We both agreed that it would be interesting to see if this would work at the dispensary. I know, this whole thing might sound weird to most people; but I was a guinea pig willing to crawl into a crop of marijuana in order to get to the bottom of this mystery.

Once I had the prescription in hand, I had to plan my visit to correlate with how well I felt. I could barely lift my head off my pillow most of the time; therefore I had to wait for the most opportune moment. I decided to go on a Monday because I didn't have radiation treatments on Saturday and Sunday. I felt the best, yet still awful, on Monday. My radiation appointment was early that day so I decided to go after the appointment. I had no idea how long it would take. Hence I made sure to dose-up on anti-nausea meds to ensure they were at peak performance levels.

Unfortunately, the day this all came together happened to fall on Barb's birthday. I had already ruined a few of her birthdays with a back injury one year and thyroid surgery another. Again, caregivers deserve such high praise for the sacrifices they must endure while taking care of a cancer patient. When all was said and done, she admitted that she'd never had a more "interesting" birthday than when we went on our adventure to secure medicinal marijuana. That's right up there with getting a pony for your birthday.

With Rx in hand, we ventured out to find the dispensary. We didn't know what to expect. Even though we had the address, we passed by it twice. In a row of non-descript, mid-century houses along a busy street we saw a beige house with nothing more than a green cross (rather than red designated for all things medical), and an "Open" sign in one of the front windows.

We pulled into a driveway leading to a parking lot behind the house. I was feeling a mix of emotions. Of course I was nauseous, but I was also curious, amused, and a bit excited at the prospect of curtailing the nausea-beast and having a great story to tell.

I got out of the car and asked Barb if she was going to go with me inside. She shook her head "no" and locked her door. We both had a chuckle, and I headed for the back door. I was especially amused at the irony of the situation because Barb used to hold the title of Substance Abuse Prevention Coordinator for a school district; and here she was, sitting in the parking lot of a pot dispensary. This stuff writes itself.

Walking up the ramp, I didn't know what to expect. As I entered the back door of the dispensary, I was hit by a waft of lingering pot aroma. No one was in the immediate lobby area; but I did hear the stereotypical cadence of a marijuana dude's voice talking on the phone. I rang a bell and a young man came out to greet me. I was expecting to hear the line from the hilarious sketch, The Californians from *Saturday Night Live*, "Uh, whaaaat are youuu doing here?"

Instead, he asked, "How may I help you?"

The prescription from my oncologist apparently wasn't considered a "recommendation." Instead, he told me I had to go to a specific doctor's office down the street where I could pay sixty dollars to get an appointment and a medicinal marijuana card. He handed me a glossy 4" x 6" coupon for a discount on the exam, and off I went. The adventure was taking a turn, but I was still in it to find a cure for my nausea.

We drove to the address listed on the coupon only to find a sign on the door in the urine-soaked alcove saying the office had moved. In case you're wondering, yes, the smell of the urine-soaked alcove made me dry heave.

Once we found our way to the new address, we parked. I got out and Barb once again locked the door. I found the almost-secret-red-door entrance. Each step of this adventure was a first; and I couldn't wait to see what the next one would bring.

The waiting room deserves some descriptive elaboration. It was a large, somewhat dingy room with pale blue walls. Approximately fifty chairs lined the walls and filled a few meandering rows. All the people in the room looked like they got kicked out of class in high school and were waiting to see the principal. No one looked sick; and everyone seemed to be in their twenties. Anyone who looked remotely like a mom, senior citizen or child was mysteriously missing. This office was absent of medical-office dignity, and I had lost my dignity many days prior.

Across the room was a counter with a glass window. I headed that way and was greeted by a man behind the window with a thick Russian accent. He told me to fill out some forms, bring them back to him, and then I would be called to see the doctor. Once the doctor gave me my "recommendation," I was to return to the window and pay my sixty dollars, get my picture taken, and be given my medicinal marijuana card.

I filled in the basic information. However, the section asking about documented medical proof of a medical condition indicated it was okay if I didn't have it. All I could think was how fraudulent this whole process seemed. Apparently, all the people around me didn't seem to have a problem with that. I was feeling like crap so I didn't either.

I waited and watched the other "patients" go into the doctor's office. Each did not spend more than five minutes getting their "recommendation." As time passed, I became increasingly nervous - not because I felt like the Feds would bust in and take me to jail and force me to submit to a cavity search in my weakened state; but because as the minutes ticked by, my anti-nausea medication was swiftly losing its minimal effect.

My name was called and I was excited to see who and what was behind the curtain. I entered the office and sat down. Across the desk from me was a slumping middle-aged portly man in a grayish-white medical coat. There was a stethoscope sitting on a ledge behind him and a couple of those plastic body part replicas. Let me just say that my set designer friend would have cringed at the unrealistic medical office vibe going on in there.

The doctor-man said, "Hello, I'm Doctor So-and-So. What brings you here today?"

I pulled out my Rx from my oncologist, handed it to him and said, "I'm in chemotherapy."

He took a couple seconds to read, "Patient is in chemotherapy. Patient may benefit from medicinal marijuana," and then he quickly filled out my "recommendation."

As we parted he said, "I hope you feel better soon."

I thanked him and said, "Me too, Doctor ...Dude."

I returned to the window to pay my fee and noticed an ornery woman sitting to the right of the window in charge of taking photos. She was arguing with the Russian behind the counter. She was relentless and loudly went on-and-on telling him how unprofessional he was. Oh how I love irony. He wasn't saying a word and was trying to focus on his job. In her mind, she was busy being "professional."

I paid my fee and I waited for the ornery woman to take my photo. She was great at multi-tasking. She continued to berate the Russian while still taking people's photos. Amazing! Once my picture was taken, I waited a couple minutes for it to develop and then got my coveted medicinal marijuana card. Funny thing, even though I felt like crap, that picture turned out better than the one I have on my driver's license. The DMV has *got* to get new cameras!

By the time we made it back to the dispensary, we were two hours in on our adventure. We got there right in time for Happy Hour. I'm not kidding. Happy Hour ran from 4:20 p.m. to 6:20 p.m. every day. The significance of 4:20 started back in the 1960's on college campuses and was designated as the time for everyone to get high. I told you I was in this to learn new things.

Prior to starting our journey that day, I read on the dispensary's website that no one was allowed in "The Bud Room" without a doctor's recommendation. What I conjured up in my mind was a room with high-tech electronically sealed glass doors where a buzzer goes off, the door unlocks, and you enter. When I returned to the dispensary the Mary Jane-Dude welcomed me back. I showed him the "recommendation," my new sixty-dollar card, and told him the address on the coupon he gave me was wrong. He said he forgot to tell me. No surprise there.

He looked at the recommendation and said, "Okay great, let's go into The Bud Room."

He literally took two steps down the hall and parted the hanging beads in the doorway and welcomed me to enter. I'd have to say that threshold of exclusivity was probably as low-tech as you can get. It was so much better in my imagination.

On one side of the room was a glass case displaying edible forms of marijuana; and on the other side were jars filled with marijuana to be smoked. I opted for the edible form because I didn't want to smoke it. The smell would have killed me. I was there to help my nausea not add to the problem. The cookies were calling my name.

Mary Jane-Dude told me it was Happy Hour so the cookies were half price: $5 instead of $10 per cookie; and if I bought two I could get the third for free. Each cookie looked like it would taste really good even though I know Mrs. Fields probably didn't lend them her cookie recipe. One peanut butter cookie, chocolate, and a cranberry-oatmeal were my choices. Dude's only instructions were not to eat any more than a quarter of a cookie at a time to see how it affected me. He gave me another coupon and advised me that they would deliver future orders to my house. That was astonishing. That would have been a pretty funny joke thirty years ago. I paid the Dude and I was out of the building.

I made it to the parking lot and stood behind our car and waved my hands so I wouldn't scare Barb by knocking on the window. She unlocked the door.

I slid in and said, "Please get me home." I put the bag of cookies in the back seat because it reeked of pot, a smell of which I was never a fan.

Our adventure took everything out of me. When I got home, I crashed on the couch. After a few minutes, I mustered the energy to cut an eighth of a piece of the peanut butter cookie. As I raised it to my mouth, the pot smell was so strong it made me gag. I put it in my mouth, chewed it like a kid being forced to eat a vegetable, washed it down with some water and returned to the couch.

Are you hoping for a happy ending like I was? The happy ending didn't come. It didn't work for me. Those familiar strange thoughts that swore me off the stuff thirty years prior were swirling in my head. My body felt sedated but the nausea was still there. I was hugely disappointed, probably just like you are right now. At least it does make for a memorable story.

Those cookies sat on the kitchen counter wrapped in plastic for the duration of my treatment. I never ate any more of my stash, and once treatment was complete, the nausea left and I threw the cookies away. This was a big disappointment for some friends, but frankly, throwing them away was part of gaining my power back. Seeing them in the trashcan and watching the trash man drive away with them in his truck was a spectacular feeling.

The nausea finally left about a week after completing treatment. The magnitude of the relief I felt was one of the best feelings I've ever had in my life. I hope to never again do time in nausea prison. The pot dispensary has since been closed so at least I know I won't be going back there.

A year later when my medicinal marijuana card expired I celebrated having the year behind me; but most importantly we gave Barb the drug-free birthday celebration she deserved.

Cн 14 - ANECDOTE FOR AN ANTIDOTE

Warning: this is the most scientific-y chapter in this book. While it may scare some of you away, let me assure you the information is fascinating, thought provoking, and makes for a great story. Additionally, for those who love science, my hope is to provide you with inspiration to further investigate the things mentioned in this chapter and to one day bring benefits to the masses. You're welcome. Don't forget to credit me in your next journal article submission.

Webster's Dictionary defines an anecdote as information that is subjective, circumstantial, hearsay, unreliable, untrustworthy, undependable, and sketchy. Whereas, an antidote is defined as a cure, remedy, solution, answer, corrective, medicine. What if the cure for cancer starts as an anecdote and develops into the antidote? Every discovery needs a starting point.

Volumes of research journals are filled with studies conducted using small groups of subjects; some of them as small as one person. Can you imagine if you were the one person who benefitted from the research? Wouldn't you want to share that benefit with everyone? Wouldn't you like to have people believe you when you tell them how great you feel having experienced the benefit of a treatment? Are you also willing to accept that fact that some doctors, dentists, nurses, friends and family are going to doubt or discount what you are saying? You should be ready for that, but don't let it deter you from your path.

Once I completed chemotherapy and radiation I knew I wanted to nurse myself back to health. I felt an overwhelming need to detox my system and set myself up for a healthy future. All my tissues felt the impact of the treatment. Fatigue was my new best-worst friend; and I had to really make an effort to roundup energy to do anything. My bloodwork showed both red and white blood cell counts were low. That meant my system was suffering from lower than normal levels of oxygen present in red blood cells; and my immune system took a huge hit resulting in lower than normal white blood cells. The veins in my arms and hands were damaged and felt bumpy along the length of the vein and in various spots where chemotherapy needles had been placed. Although others said I looked good, I knew I didn't. At least I didn't feel like I looked anywhere close to good. However, I was elated the sickly suffering was gone. I've said it before and I'll say it again: relentless nausea was the hardest most debilitating aspect of the entire journey.

I knew better than to expect my M.D.s or my healthcare insurance providers to help me with the rejuvenation part of my journey. It's not really in their wheelhouse of skills and services. The investment of time and money you put into your own rejuvenation will be the best money you have ever spent. You're worth it – period.

That being said, a friend of mine referred me to a naturopathic doctor (N.D.) who had great success with helping patients "detox" their bodies after chemotherapy. I made my first appointment with Dr. S in Costa Mesa, CA and looked forward to getting some help.

The first order of business was to determine a baseline measure of the amount of platinum still present in my system from the Cisplatin chemotherapy drug. This involved obtaining a measure directly from a urine sample collected over a six hour period. The sample was sent to an independent diagnostic lab (The Genova Diagnostic, Inc.) for analysis to determine the presence of the following toxic elements: lead, mercury, aluminum, antimony, arsenic, barium bismuth, cadmium, cesium, gadolinium, gallium, nickel, niobium, platinum, rubidium, thallium, thorium, tin, tungsten, uranium.

The initial results indicated platinum (from the Cisplatin) levels measuring 46.379 in comparison to a reference range (representative of a healthy population) of less than or equal to 0.033. My level was **1405.2 times higher** than the reference range. Please keep in mind that I was told by my oncologist that the Cisplatin would be out of my system within a few days after each treatment. This sample was taken in September 2012 - five months after my final Cisplatin treatment. My body still had **one-thousand, four-hundred and five times more platinum in my body in comparison with a healthy population!** The fact that scientific evidence showed my body was still toxic with platinum convinced me that I was given incorrect and incomplete information. Is this a result of a lack of education? Is it a sign of limited thinking about the ramifications of chemotherapy? Or sadly, is a blind eye turned so insurance companies won't have to pay claims and settle law suits? In my situation, I felt these were relevant questions; but the answers were elusive and some questions will never be answered. Most importantly, I felt that this information was crucial for me, the patient, to know so I could address the matter and rid my body of this toxin.

The narrative portion of the report indicated excessive platinum in food or drink is rare; and most exposures are industrial via inhalation, or as a result of the administration of "cis-platin", a chemotherapeutic agent for cancer (that's me). Elemental platinum has a very low toxicity except for those who have dermal sensitivity. Most inhaled, ingested or injected platinum is excreted via urine. This excretion is biphasic with most being eliminated within several hours while the remainder may require twelve days or more for excretion (in my case a lot longer). This raises the question: why is my body holding on to it?

Platinum as a complex can up-regulate heme oxygenase activity (>10x), thereby disordering heme synthesis in the liver. Platinum inhibits DNA synthesis in the same manner that it exerts its antitumor activity. Binding to and blocking sulfhydryl sites and inhibition of dehydrogenase enzymes are other modes of toxicity. Platinum deposits in the liver and in the kidney, where chronic deposition can damage proximal tubules and cause renal insufficiency. "Platinosis" caused by chronic exposure features rhinorrhea, coughing and sneezing, eczematous dermatitis, and a lung syndrome with dyspnea, wheezing and an asthma-like condition.

Besides cisplatin, sources of platinum include: catalytic converters on gasoline engines, electroplating operations, catalyst production and catalytic equipment in the chemical process industries and petroleum refineries, precious dental materials, jewelry, smelting and refining of nickel and copper, purification of gold ores, and electronic parts such as thermocouples, resistance wires and contacts.

The lab reports this level of platinum as being TMPL, Tentative Maximum Permissible Limit, meaning the element excretion is significantly elevated, consistent with increased *body burden*. Increased element concentrations can have a negative impact on overall health and well-being. These values are derived from Casaret and Doull's – Toxicology: The Basic Science of Poisons, 5th Ed, 1996 McGraw Hill New York, NY, p 997-998. The units have been standardized.

Although there were slight elevations of lead and mercury in the same sample, they, along with all other toxic elements were within the reference range. This was an indication that I was not currently being exposed to heavy metals in my environment. However, heavy metals can be stored in body tissues and bones where they can continue to cause harm.

Dr. S devised a plan to address removal of the platinum. The plan of action entailed my participation in a chelation process designed to pull the platinum and other toxic elements out of my body. The next step involved obtaining a measure of the same elements; but this time we would be using a provoking agent. I was given a kit to take home which entailed taking a heavy metal chelating agent (Meso-2, 3-dimercaptosuccinic acid - DMSA), gathering my urine for six hours and sending it off to the same independent lab for analysis.

DMSA is a compound approved in the 1960's by the FDA for the removal (chelation) of heavy metals. DMSA is considered the preferred agent in both adults and children.

The results of the *provoked* heavy metals test showed that I had 2206.1 times the amount of platinum in my system in comparison with the reference range comprised from the healthy population.

To my surprise, the test also revealed extremely high levels of lead and mercury. In fact, they were the highest levels Dr. S had seen in fifteen years of practice. It is unclear exactly when and how I had been exposed to lead and mercury in the past. I remember breaking a thermometer when I was a kid after I heated it up to fake a fever and get out of going to school. When I saw the thermometer read 104 degrees, I shook it; hit the door knob, it shattered, and mercury went everywhere. I picked up the shiny liquid globules as best I could, and was completely clueless about its toxicity.

Also, my family vacationed most summers in southern Utah during the late 1960's when the government was still conducting above-ground nuclear bomb testing in the Nevada desert. We basically vacationed in toxic clouds that traveled over southern Utah, Nevada and Arizona. Those clouds polluted land used to live upon and grow food. We always thought corn-on-the-cob at the Utah Iron County Fair tasted so good. Little did we know? All of this is well-documented, and subsequent reparations were paid by the U.S. Government to a group known as, "The Downwinders," that is until the funds dried up. Many of my relatives suffered various cancers and have either died or are currently fighting it as a result of this horrendous human-testing blunder. Even their livestock were killed and suffered birth defects.

Perhaps my high heavy metal levels had to do with my body's inability to rid itself of toxins. Maybe my system holds on to things longer in comparison with the majority whose metabolism pumps out poison better and quicker than mine. My family has a history of thyroid disease; and the thyroid gland regulates metabolism. Therefore, this may lend evidence to the notion that toxins get clogged in my system. Also, I had an uncle who suffered from Wilson's disease that caused an unhealthy accumulation of copper in his system. Our family may be magnetic to metals. Is that possible? It's worth investigating.

My lead levels measured at 51.9 with a reference range of less than or equal to 1.4, which is 37.07 times the reference range comprised from the healthy population.

I was never one of those kids who ate leaded paint chips off the window sill, or had a cluster of lead pencil tips stuck in my hand from elementary school. There is information in the literature that suggests chemotherapy works at the bone marrow level; and humans store lead in bones. As the chemotherapy disturbs the bones, lead may be releasing into a patient's system. Knowing for certain where the lead in my system came from is part of a mystery that I will likely never solve. What I do know is that I would like to get it out of my system.

According to the lab report, 70 percent to 80 percent of absorbed lead is typically excreted via urine, 15 percent to 20 percent via bile, and the remainder via sweat, hair and nails. In non-provoked urine, lead levels can fluctuate according to variable dietary and physiological factors, and the level does not necessarily reflect body burden. Provoked levels, however, can be indicative of excess lead in body tissues. It is notable that for children (compared with adults) lead can be more toxic, with detrimental effects occurring at much lower levels. Furthermore, toxicity of lead can be significantly increased synergistically by the presence of either mercury or cadmium.

Additionally, most lead uptake occurs via ingestion of contaminated food or water. Inhalation of lead dusts and transdermal absorption of organic lead salts are other modes of uptake. While temporarily carried in the bloodstream, lead is at least 90 percent bound to erythrocytes (contains the red pigment hemoglobin and transports oxygen and carbon dioxide to and from the tissues). However, with chronic low-level or long-ago exposure, only 2 percent or less of total body lead remains in the blood. Lead primarily deposits and accumulates in the aorta, liver, kidneys, adrenal and thyroid glands, bones and teeth. This element interferes with membrane functions, bonds to sulfhydryl (-SH), phosphate, hydroxyl and amino sites on proteins and enzyme cofactors, and interferes with heme synthesis, iron transport, erythrocyte life span, and hepatic cytochrome P-450 functions. Other deleterious effects include: reduced vitamin D synthesis, slowed nerve conduction, peripheral neuropathy, hypertension (adults) and loss of IQ and developmental disorders (children). Anemia (not enough red blood cells), neuropathies (damage to nerves in the peripheral nervous system), and encephalopathy (any degenerative disease of the brain), are end-stage conditions of severe lead excess.

Lastly, although historic uses of lead (house paint, anti-knock gasoline additives, and soldering joints in water systems) have been discontinued, old building materials, paint chips, plumbing and the environment may contain residual amounts from these sources. Other sources include batteries in cars, trucks, boats, and power backup systems, art supplies, colored glass kits, bullets, fishing sinkers, balance weights, radiation shields, bearing alloys, Babbitt metal (any of several alloys used for the bearing surface in a plain bearing), some ceramic glazes or pigments, and sewage sludge. Some cities that have not replaced old water mains may have variable amounts of lead in the drinking water.

Mercury is considered to be the second most toxic substance on the planet; and negative effects of mercury exposure are well documented. Uranium is the number one most toxic substance. Mercury exposure, like radiation, accumulates over time. **There are NO SAFE LEVELS for mercury in the body**. My mercury levels were 30.07 with a reference range of less than or equal to 2.19, which is **13.7 times the reference range** comprised from the healthy population.

According to the lab report, mercury behaves differently in different body tissues depending on its chemical form; and interchange between forms can occur in vivo (within living organisms, humans, animals). For elemental and inorganic mercury, biliary (relating to bile, bile ducts, or gallbladder) excretion predominates with low-level toxicity, but urinary excretion increases and is favored as the degree of exposure and burden increases. Regarding organic mercury (methyl, ethyl, alkyl), bile accounts for about ninety percent of excretion and urine accounts for about ten percent. Significant day-to-day and diurnal variations are typically observed. Urinary excretion of mercury is notably increased following administration of chelating or detoxifying agents (DMSA, DMPS); intravenous administration of EDTA results in relatively minor urinary increases. The Genova Diagnostic Inc. laboratory procedure measures total urine mercury, regardless of chemical form, and the procedure is not hindered by tightly-bound sulfhydryl-mercury that might be unavailable (and unmeasured) by the old standard procedure ("cold-vapor atomic absorption").

The report goes on to say, there is great variability in individual tolerances to mercury. In some individuals, relatively low levels can cause immune dysregulation. Lymphocyte inhibition and dysfunction is reported, immunosuppression can occur, and autoimmune conditions (I've got Hashimoto's autoimmune thyroiditis) are documented in animals. At the cellular level, mercury can induce cytotoxicity, oxidative stress (via loss of glutathione function), and increased secretion of beta-amyloid in neuronal cells, linking it to Alzheimer's disease. Outside cells, mercury can bind to and strongly inhibit a cell surface-bound protein called dipeptidylpeptidase IV, CD26, and adenosine deaminase binding protein. This one protein is responsible for digestion of proline-containing dietary peptides, T-cell activation, and the metabolism of adenosine. Inside cells, mercury binds to lipoic acid, glutathione, coenzyme A and cysteinyl sites, and it can impair pyruvate metabolism and citric acid (Krebs) cycle function, leading to impaired energy production. Chronic mercury exposure may produce increased excitability and tremor, memory loss, insomnia, lassitude, anorexia and weight loss, gingivitis and stomatitis. Young children may exhibit "pink disease" (acrodynia), commonly featuring rash, photophobia, increased perspiration and salivation. Acute mercury vapor exposure may inflame the bronchial tubes and cause pneumonitis. Irreversible neurological damage is reported in acute mercury toxicity. Inorganic mercury concentrates mostly in kidneys, while organic (methyl) mercury has high affinity for the posterior cortex of the brain.

Finally, mercury sources have increased in the environment, resulting in increased amounts in soils, sediments and bodies of water. Coal-fired power plants emit over 30 percent of environmentally released mercury. Other industrial sources are chlorine or "chlor-alkali" plants, cement plants, pulp and paper mills, municipal waste incinerators (19 percent of total release), and hazardous/medical waste incinerators. As of 2001, over 100 tons of mercury is "missing" from the EPA-surveyed inventory of chlor-alkali plants which admit to releasing the element to air and landfills. These sources, along with increased farming, forest fires, mining and excavations, and volcanoes, have served to increase surface deposition (micrograms per square meter) of mercury in surveyed areas by over 300 percent since 1850. This mercury can be biologically changed into organic forms and made bioavailable. Fish, shellfish and edible seaweed then become dietary sources of this element. Other sources include: old latex paint (manufactured before 1990), antifungal and antifouling (marine) paints, some fluorescent light tubes and vapor lamps, medicinal products such as those containing "Thimerosal" (sodium ethyl mercurithiosalicylate or mercurothiolate—often contained in routine vaccines), explosives and detonators, batteries and "calomel" electrodes, electrical switches, thermostats and relays, and scientific or laboratory equipment (thermometers, barometers). Dental amalgams are primarily a source of elemental or amalgamated mercury that is typically found in feces for several days following dental procedures; very little of this dental-procedure mercury appears in urine. However, mercury vapor from in-place amalgam fillings can be absorbed, bio-transformed and excreted in urine, but its level is typically much less than that which is attributable to food sources, especially seafood.

The lab test results showed that all other levels of toxic elements were within the reference range.

Platinum, lead and mercury were identified as the formidable opponents for my chelation program. Dr. S laid out a plan for me to follow:

1. I would take 500 mg of DSMA as a chelating agent twice a day for three days.
2. Take ten days off.
3. Repeat.

He told me that the process can take quite a long time; but as long as repeated test results showed improvement, we would continue the program until my platinum, lead and mercury levels returned to a healthy reference range. I told him I was in it for the long haul if that's what it took. Some adjustments were made to my dosage overtime and I settled into a routine of taking 500 mg of DSMA twice a day for two days, with seven days off. We periodically retested my urine to obtain measures of progress.

An unsettling event happened after I underwent an MRI on March 7, 2013 to scan my liver, which included a contrast agent called, gadolinium (a toxic element). If you recall, prior to surgery my PET scan showed there was something, other than cancer, going on in my liver. It was on the "to do" list to investigate this further. In my heavy metal urine test collected on March 28, 2013 levels of gadolinium were measured at 46.68 with a reference range of less than or equal to 0.019, which is **2457.1 times the reference range comprised from the healthy population.** Unfortunately, this test also surprisingly showed that both my mercury and lead levels had doubled in comparison to a test sample collected on December 26, 2012 (Mercury - 16.32 increased to 34.51; Lead - 12.2 increased to 23.9). This was a setback; and I was upset because I was not told about the type of contrast agent being used in the MRI; but then again, I didn't realize it was a problem until after the metal test. When I stepped out of the MRI room I did ask the MRI tech what was used as the contrast agent. He told me it was gadolinium. I usually ask that question with any scan I have to ensure iodine is not used, which may cause harm to my already-compromised half-of-a-thyroid gland. Once I got the metal test results, I went home and researched gadolinium. I learned that there is controversy surrounding this contrast agent, which has caused problems for some people. The unfortunate thing is that research indicated there are alternative contrasting agents to be used for people who have sensitivities; but it was too late for me. I'm completely, utterly frustrated because I cannot be expected to know everything about every procedure before I have it. Ugh!

According to the lab report, gadolinium is a member of a group of rare earth metals known as lanthanides. It has been used for superconductors, magnets, fluorescent materials, and as a nuclear MRI contrast agent. Toxicity appears similar to nickel and copper, and has been associated with hair loss and skin lesions. These changes are consistent with zinc deficiency and are correlated with increased urinary zinc concentrations.

I later discovered a journal article titled, Toxic Effects of Mercury, Lead and Gadolinium on Vascular Reactivity (Brazilian Journal of Medical and Biological Research (2011) 44: 939-946). The results of the study suggest that mercury, lead and gadolinium, even at low doses or concentrations, affect vascular reactivity. Acting via the endothelium, by continuous exposure followed by their absorption, they can increase the production of free radicals and of angiotensin II, representing a hazard for cardiovascular function. In addition, the actual reference values noted in the study, considered to pose no risk, need to be reduced. You can imagine my upset when I read this article. My body was already burdened with platinum, mercury, lead, and now gadolinium was coursing through my body.

To top it all off, the results of the MRI showed I have small cysts throughout my liver known as Von Meyenburg Complexes (VCMs): a rare pathologic entity, consisting of small (<1.5 cm), usually multiple and nodular cystic lesions. VCMs typically cause no symptoms or disturbances in liver function and thus in most instances they are diagnosed incidentally. Although these are apparently benign, I had reason to be concerned. When I was diagnosed with cancer my sister, Lisa decided to do some family research on ancestry.com. She discovered that my Great

Aunt Ruby, who I never knew, died from uterine cancer in 1951. This was before the Pap test was even invented, and radiation therapy was just becoming available. I don't think she ever stood a chance. The secondary cause of death listed on the death certificate was cirrhosis of the liver. Aunt Ruby was a stanch non-drinker so I'm assuming it was the non-alcoholic cirrhosis variety. I'll never know if the person performing the autopsy wrote down cirrhosis when in fact it may have been Von Meyenburg Complexes. Yikes! Or visa-versa – do I really have cirrhosis of the liver? For my own sanity, I'm sticking with my benign VCM diagnosis for now. In my mind I wondered if I inherited Aunt Ruby's internal organs. This is a perfect example of the importance of doing genealogy work to determine your hereditary health risks. My father never allowed us to locate his father's side of the family; but now there's ancestry.com and the information is available.

All I could do was put my blinders on and continue with my regime to rid my body of these toxins. To date, I've had significant improvements in my levels, which are noted in the table below:

HEAVY METAL	TEST DATE	8/28/12	12/26/12	3/28/13	1/16/14	9/9/14
PLATINUM		72.8	31.85	23.2	10.35	6.036
LEAD		51.9	12.2	23.9	22.4	30.5*
MERCURY		30.07	16.32	34.5	17.34	15.95
GADOLINIUM		N/A	N/A	46.68	0.31	0.166

Note: * Increase in lead in 9/9/14 test results may or may not be attributed to increased bone loss, which may or may not be related to hormonal depletion subsequent to radical hysterectomy to remove cervical cancer. Results of a bone density test are pending.

Based on the test results covering the period August 28, 2012 to September 9, 2014 (24 months) I have seen a 92 percent reduction in platinum, a 53 percent reduction in lead, a 47 percent reduction in mercury, and a 99.6 percent reduction in gadolinium.

These numbers should impress anyone who is the slightest bit interested in the potential benefit chelation programs hold for chemotherapy patients. Yes, I realize that I am a sample size of one; but remember all antidotes start with an anecdote. If anything, this provides information for those who seek new frontiers in medicine.

This is as good a time as any to tell you that for nine years I experienced pain and numbness on the right side of my face including in my ear, jaw, down into my neck, in my tongue, inside my throat, and my eye and eyelid. The question as to how my mercury levels got so high in the first place was a topic of discussion and intrigue during my visits with Dr. S. He suspected that the pain in my face may be due to two mercury amalgam fillings in two teeth in the upper right side of my mouth. I have been lucky to only have one dental cavity in my life, and one of the two fillings was due to that cavity. The other small filling was placed at the outer most edge of my last molar because the edge of the tooth had been chipped, was sharp and causing problems.

The issue of mercury's negative effects is contentious for some dentists. The CDC (United States Centers for Disease Control and Prevention) indicates that amalgam fillings are comprised of 50 percent metallic mercury, 35 percent silver, 9 percent tin, 6 percent copper and trace amounts of zinc. They also state the following about amalgam fillings: further study is needed to determine the possibility of behavioral or immune system effects, and to determine the levels of exposure that may lead to adverse effects in sensitive populations. Sensitive populations may include pregnant women, children under that age of six years, people with impaired kidney function, and people with hypersensitive immune responses to metals. Do your research and join in on the controversy. I'm committed to faulting on the side of safety rather than ignorantly holding on to a belief that might cause cancer to recur. It's not even up for discussion.

In 2008 I had a right side thyroidectomy due to a tangerine size nodule on the thyroid gland. Prior to surgery I was experiencing right side facial pain and thought perhaps it was the nodule pressing on nerves. There are so many nerves in the neck and head that it was a reasonable probability. Once I recovered from surgery, the pain was still present. At the direction of my surgeon, and a neurologist I underwent multiple scans that eventually determined my condition was idiopathic: the cause was not readily apparent.

The pain in my tongue alone felt like someone constantly squeezing it. It always felt like it was in a cramp. Don't be surprised if you suddenly become hyperaware of your tongue right now. When I opened my mouth I could see that my tongue sat unevenly in my mouth. Toward the back of my throat where my uvula is, the right side arch drooped down and did not move up when saying, "Ah" like it did on the left side. I had difficulty swallowing and increasingly had difficulty pronouncing some words. I even began slurring words. My ability to swallow was affected. Sometimes liquid would not go all the way down my throat when I swallowed. It would involuntarily find its way into my throat and I would choke and cough. I described the feeling to the doctor as feeling like a flat spot in my tongue that didn't follow the usual wave-like motion which occurs during a normal swallow. Try it. Isn't your tongue amazing?

My jaw was always aching and I endured multiple chiropractic adjustments to my Temporal-mandibular joint (TMJ). I also endured acupuncture in my tongue. Yes, needles in my tongue, multiple times. I consulted with my dentist at the time who told me there was nothing wrong with my trigeminal nerve that innervates some areas where I was having pain. After many years attempting to get relief, I finally gave up. What else could I do? When a medical community tells you there is no known cause, and they look at you funny, it shuts you down. That is until I met Dr. S; and yes, until I had cervical cancer.

Dr. S suggested that I get my amalgam filling removed. He also recommended that I watch "Smoking Teeth" on YouTube (Link to watch it yourself: https://www.youtube.com/watch?v=9ylnQ-T7oiA) to see evidence of mercury gasses escaping from teeth fillings. Although you can't believe everything you see on YouTube, this video is extremely thought-provoking. He was confident that removal of the filling would make a big difference. Not only would a legitimate source of mercury be eliminated from my body, but he was optimistic that I might see improvement in the facial, tongue, eye and jaw pain I had been experiencing for nine years. The anticipation alone was so exhilarating.

Initially, I went to my dentist to have the filling removed. At that time I thought I had only one filling. Dr. B, my dentist, removed the filling on November 1, 2012 and replaced it with a white, resin-composite filling. He also told me that there was no "scientific proof" that mercury would affect anyone negatively. I let him believe that because he was about sixty days away from retiring. I think that is such an ignorant and damaging thing to tell a patient. He didn't know I had been well-educated in the methods and practices of scientific research. "Scientific proof" is a squirrely phrase that some use to posture their case and defend a position on an issue. My instructors always warned me about those who use research statistics to influence others in a way that plays on people's lack of knowledge on the matter. First and foremost, research never "proves" anything; but rather, the tests show levels of significance for the sample being tested.

Dr. B removed the filling without taking the precaution of using a dental dam, which I found out later was highly recommended to avoid exposing the patient to more mercury. Not only did he neglect to use a dental dam, but six months later I removed a small chunk of amalgam filling embedded in my tonsil. How disgustingly crazy is that, and who knows what damage that caused? The nerves that innervate the tonsil run up into the sinus area and into the eye, which happened to be the remaining area where I have pain. I'm never going to turn this into a litigious legal matter; but my story could help someone prevent their own health problems.

I know plenty of people who experience multiple sensitivities. A friend of mine was allergic to the metal in the partial bridge holding her two false front teeth in place. She endured years of irritated gums and pain. It wasn't until she went to a new female dentist who determined she was in fact allergic to the metal in her dental work. This is a prime example of a patient experiencing adverse reactions to metal. There are many other examples in the research. Some dentists still hold on to their "rightness" while the patient is told incorrect and extremely harmful information. I will never understand that!

A small second filling was removed July 31, 2013. The reason for the delay was the fact that I didn't realize the filling was amalgam. I thought Dr. B had used a bonding agent to fill the small portion of my tooth that had cracked off. I might sound ignorant for not knowing this, but it was in the upper back part of my tooth that could only be seen with a mirror placed inside my mouth. By the time I realized it was there, Dr. B had retired. It was safely removed by Dr. N, my new, more forward-thinking dentist, who bought Dr. B's dental practice. Dr. N took all the proper precautions to protect me from mercury exposure. He also told me that he had removed other people's fillings and some had benefitted; others had not. I was relieved to have both fillings removed, and excited to see if my facial pain would improve.

In what I consider nothing short of a miracle, slowly but surely over the next year the pain faded. First, my jaw stopped aching. Then my tongue didn't hurt; and any tendency to slur my words disappeared. Swallowing liquids was effortless once again. At the time of writing this book, the only pain that remains is a small area around my eye, the inner corner of my eyelid; and I still have pain inside my eyeball. When it's cold and breezy my eye area, ear and neck are sensitive. I'm hoping all the pain resolves soon; but I realize it may be permanent.

Imagine having a constant, relentless pain in your face, jaw, tongue and neck for nine years. Then a naturopathic doctor helps you discover a cure through scientifically analyzing the heavy metal burden in your body after chemotherapy! We were looking for Cisplatin levels and stumbled across some mercury that was the cause of all my pain. I am brought to tears just thinking about it. Mystery solved, and now we know my condition was **not idiopathic.**

I'm not the only one to experience these results. Do your research and you will see that many people are finding a way to return to better health by eliminating amalgam fillings from their mouth. You will also continue to read about dentists who still don't believe any of it. What do they stand to lose by admitting there is a problem? Unfortunately, the answer is likely, money by way of litigation.

My best advice during the period of recovery and rejuvenation is to be informed and keep good records. You are the conductor of your own case study. Read as much as you can. Scrutinize articles from respected journals, university-based books, and internet information with a keen eye. Check sources and valid measures of correctness. Doctors don't know everything. That's not a putdown; it's just an impossible expectation to place upon them. They simply don't have time to read every journal article published if they are seeing eighty to one-hundred patients or more a day and barely get time to eat. I've been known to hand-carry an article in and give my doctor a copy to have for my file.

It's my responsibility to keep them informed of things that impact my treatment.

On one such occasion I went to the ophthalmologist because I had a problem with my right eye, in addition to the pain I was already having as noted above. One night I was outside and I would quickly look to the right and left and I would see flashes of light that looked like lightening along the outer edges of my eye. The darkness of night made it much more obvious. It scared the hell out of me because I remembered the movie, *Phenomenon*, in which John Travolta played a guy who saw a flash in the sky one night. Cut to: it ended up being a brain tumor. Yes, when you have had cancer you have a tendency to escalate everything to a worst-case scenario. I'd never had this kind of thing happen before. At minimum, I wondered if I was going blind or having a stroke. Fortunately none of these self-diagnoses were correct.

It was time to make an appointment with the ophthalmologist to find out what was going on. Prior to going to the appointment I researched my symptoms. I found an article in the Journal of Cancer Therapeutics & Research titled, Ocular Adverse Effects of Anti-cancer Chemotherapy and Targeted Therapy, authored by Parul Singh and Abhishek Singh, available through HOAJ (Herbert Open Access Journals). The article states that ocular toxicity induced by anti-cancer chemotherapy is not uncommon, but underestimated and under-reported. Visual changes have been attributed to a number of chemotherapeutic agents including my chemo drug Cisplatin. According to the article, Cisplatin is known to produce non-specific blurred vision, papilledema, unilateral as well as bilateral retro bulbar neuritis and optic neuritis, transient cortical blindness, temporary homonymous hemianopia, macular pigmentary changes. It goes on to mention another study in which thirteen women were treated with cisplatin for ovarian tumors. Eight of them developed blurred vision, three developed decreased color vision, six patients reported irregular pigmentation in the macula, and nine experienced cone dysfunction on electro-retinogram (ERG).

I was excited to share this information with the ophthalmologist in hopes that it would increase the quality of my visit and eventual treatment. The more information, the better.

By the time I had the appointment, the flashes of light had lessened; but a huge blurry blob of something was floating inside my eyeball, and two rows of black hairy floaters crisscrossed my field of vision like I was watching my own personal motion-graphics show. It was, and still is awful to deal with and makes me feel dizzy and off-balance.

I went to my appointment and told the doctor about "the whole cancer thing" and shared the article with him. Platinum was still present in my system based on my lab work and he didn't believe that had anything to do with my symptoms. He did NOT want a copy of the article and he basically "poo-pooed" me. He chalked my problem (possible posterior vitreous detachment) up to age, which made me extremely mad. It's a shame. He lost out on the potential of discovering something that could help thousands of people if he had just taken more of an interest in my case. Ironically, the article I wanted to give him mentions the *under-reporting* of ocular problems due to chemotherapeutic agents; and here he was turning away from an opportunity to report my problem to someone who might be able to do something about it.

No one likes to be minimized, especially people still recovering from cancer treatment. I left there feeling defeated because not only did he not listen to me, he also told me there was nothing to be done about my condition. That's not the first time I've heard that. He just gave me some eye drops which contained a preservative I'm not supposed to have, and told me to come back in two weeks. Yeah, I didn't go back. The biggest bummer is that I just bought a full 1080 HD computer screen; and I'll likely never get to truly appreciate the beauty of the awesome Ultra 4K HD TVs of today. Seriously though, our vision is such a blessing. I'm a very "visual person" so to have these problems really bums me out. The gifts that cancer gives just keep coming.

That experience convinced me that I needed to find another ophthalmologist - one that may help me resolve the permanent blurry blob floating inside my eyeball. Perhaps I'll start with the doctors who authored the research study mentioned above. I want to find someone who will take an interest in my case and accept an article from a patient's outstretched hand, even if we never find a cure for the problem.

I have discovered that some doctors from different disciplines often times disregard practitioners in other healing professions. I am responsible to educate myself on ways to wade through information guiding my healthcare, and how to stay out of the fray between M.D.s, Chiropractors, Naturopaths, Herbalists,

Acupuncturist, and even the Pot-Doc affiliated with medicinal marijuana dispensaries.

I learned to welcome all information and determine what is best for my situation. I have good and bad stories about all of the above-mentioned healthcare professionals. There are no guarantees when it comes to healthcare providers. I cannot expect it to be otherwise. When I find a good one, I fight hard to keep him or her like I would for a great plumber, electrician or contractor who arrives on time.

Call me strange, but I really enjoyed the five statistics classes that I was required to take for my B.A. degree in psychology and my M.S. degree in counseling. Most people aren't fans of statistics. I'm pretty comfortable with understanding statistics and how they are used in research. My comfort allows me to mitigate my upset when research results are discounted or dismissed for one reason or another. I just brush it off and continue to believe there should be more research done so others could benefit.

The cancer journey has steered me toward some relevant questions that could be the source for groundbreaking research. The fact that Alzheimer's disease has ruined my mom's life, and that she had chemotherapy might have something to do with the formulation of these questions:

1. Do people who have had chemotherapy have an increased chance of getting Alzheimer's disease due to the lead and other metals being released into the body from storage in the bone?

2. Do people who have had chemotherapy and refrain from hormone replacement to avoid recurrence have a higher likelihood of getting Alzheimer's disease due to bone degeneration (osteoporosis) and release of stored lead from the bones?

3. Is "Chemo-brain" a result of stored toxins and lead and mercury; and should efforts be made to remove it from all chemo patients after completion of treatment to avoid neurological, cognitive problems and potential for developing Alzheimer's disease?

And an extra credit question:

4. I have Hashimoto's thyroiditis, an autoimmune disease that destroys the thyroid gland due to increased thyroid antibody activity. It has been 34 months since my final chemotherapy treatment and my white blood cell count remains lower than the normal range. Since undergoing chemo, my blood work shows a huge decrease in thyroid antibodies which were 1900 (as high as 2100) before chemo. Although a normal level of thyroid antibodies should be <30, mine of late measure 54. This decrease is substantial and raises the question: has chemotherapy slowed the progression of the Hashimoto's? Could this help find a new treatment for this endocrine disease?

You may never hear someone say, "If I had to do the whole cancer thing again I would..." Well, I definitely don't want to do it again; but if the clock turned back and I knew what I now know, I would definitely gather a lot of pre-test data on the physical and psychological variables that have come into question for me.

Based on what I experienced and from what I see happen to others, I believe great things would be learned if pre-tests and post-tests were set up to measure the following:

1. The levels of heavy metals in a person's body. The presence of mercury, lead, gadolinium, platinum, uranium, etc. in a person's system could be measured and addressed before chemotherapy and after. I was told that the platinum in Cisplatin would clear out of my system in a short amount of time. I've got scientific evidence that shows two years and eight months after the completion of my chemotherapy that my lab results are still showing levels of platinum. The presence of platinum causes DNA changes that are detrimental to health and recovery. Cancer and various other neurological and cognitive difficulties can be caused by the presence of heavy metals. The warnings are always focused more heavily on children because they are developing. Aren't we *developing* adults? Don't we want to live a healthy life? We must focus on the adults who are being damaged by these heavy metal toxins. For some reason American western medicine refrains from addressing these things unlike many other countries that not only acknowledge the impact of such toxins, but include it in routine medical care.

2. A person's cognitive abilities, problem solving, memory etc. Subjective reports are the only thing most of us have to know for sure if our mental abilities have been negatively impacted. Without supporting evidence these issues cannot get addressed and will likely be dismissed by doctors and insurance companies.

3. Levels of a person's anxiety. Fear finds its way into a patient's mind and accelerates due to a loss of control over one's life and the situation at hand. It would provide vital information to the patient and others to determine if and when help is needed.

4. Levels of a person's depression. It is common for patients to get depressed about their situation and life in general. Many patients experience post-traumatic stress disorder symptoms that do not get addressed. This information would enhance a person's self-awareness and guide treatment if necessary.

5. A person's beliefs about body image. Surgery, chemotherapy and radiation inflict damage upon our physical body, which needs to be addressed and resolved. Some will suffer more than others depending on how they viewed themselves before diagnosis. Everyone suffers some form of loss and subsequent grief for the physical and emotional being they were before cancer. Unfortunately, there is the challenge of creating a shift in how one thinks and feels about one's body. You may struggle to find a way to shift from feeling disgusted about your body. This shift must occur in your own head and heart if you ever expect to find resolve. The simple wisdom is to be kind to yourself and purposefully engage in those things that allow it to happen.

6. A person's locus of control: a psychological concept that refers to how strongly people believe they have control over the situation and experiences that affect their lives. Does the person generally feel like they are in control of their life before diagnosis, or does the outside world control them? How does it change after the process? How do you get your power back if you believe you have lost it?

7. A person's belief in the existence of a higher power. Does a person believe in a higher power source that can unburden them of their troubling thoughts and stress? How does that change after the process?

8. A person's overall quality of life. If a person was unhappy in life to begin with, how has it changed? Also, if a person was happy and is now unhappy, what can be done to help? It is important to determine how life was going for a patient at the time of diagnosis. Personally, I had very little income at the time of diagnosis and was trying to find more dependable work. The industry in which I counseled people had pretty much been eliminated a few years ago, which was the impetus for my efforts to make a living as a freelance writer. I was two years in on my big plan when the recession hit, and I'm still suffering. Making matters worse, my mother was sliding downhill into the abyss of Alzheimer's; and I was the sibling most closely responsible for helping her. I realize that cancer never comes along at a good time for anyone. I think it would help the course of treatment if all those who provide care to cancer patients were aware of the pile of crap upon which the cancer was heaped.

9. A person's level of education and understanding about loss and the grieving process. Most people are taught how to acquire things; but little is ever taught about losing something or someone. Cancer creates a substantial amount of loss in one's life: loss of physical capacity, loss of trust, loss of safety, loss of family, loss of mental capacity, loss of purpose, etc. Friends, family and caregivers experience grief during the process as well. Whether you are the patient, friend, family or caregiver, one must educate oneself and be able to recognize the symptoms of unresolved grief, which can manifest in various types of behavior.

Funding will always be an issue, but wouldn't it be great if the post tests could be taken at three to six month intervals following treatment for five years - even ten years. The way I see it, follow-up will continue your entire life. It's a given. Realistically, there will always be the potential for receiving that tap on the shoulder to step out of life. This is a truth we share with everyone because that potential is always there whether you've had cancer or not.

The probability that an insurance company or other entity will pay for any of the research is highly unlikely; but there's always Kickstarter and Indiegogo. This doesn't wipe away the importance of addressing these issues. For me, working on each of them has been part of my quest toward finding peace, which is allowing me to have a more joyful life.

I'm excited to see more positive outcomes while I continue on my heavy metal chelation program. I'll remain guardedly optimistic that I will get my numbers down to a healthy range. That's my goal and I'm sticking to it because my anecdotal, empirically derived results may lead to the antidote for cancer, a disease that everyone must try to understand if we hope to save lives.

Cʜ 15 - 101 "MUST HAVE" SURVIVAL TIPS FOR THE WHOLE CANCER THING

In no particular order:

1.   People are going to say stupid things to you.

2.   Doctors are specialists for individual body parts so you must be the one to monitor ALL of your body parts. Don't forget any.

3.   You are the leader and team captain of your health care.

4.   Expect some people to stay a safe distance away from your struggle, but do what you can to lessen that distance and bring them back into your life as soon as you are ready.

5.   Appreciate everyone that helps you and tell them so as often as possible.

6.   You will be afraid, but you will develop skills or a good drug combination to handle that fear.

7.   Keep notes during the entire process, including the items discussed during every doctor's appointment. Always bring a pad of paper and a pen, or electronic gadget to your appointments.

8. The medical bills will pile up, but they do make for really great kindling for a cozy fire in the fireplace once they are paid, or not.

9. People will treat you differently, which is okay.

10. Appreciate every moment you are not barfing.

11. Thank the healthcare workers that are really helpful, and tattle on the ones who aren't.

12. You may develop a tendency to cuss more than usual, or for the first time, during the cancer journey.

13. You will count Mondays to get you through the waiting, but be assured that time will always move along.

14. If you are against tattoos you will have to change your mind about them if you must undergo radiation treatments.

15. Speak up for yourself, or get someone to do it for you.

16. Do not suffer in silence.

17. Give flowers, candy and lots of kindness to your caregiver during the journey and for the rest of your life. They deserve it.

18. Marijuana is likely available for those who need it during their cancer journey, even though it is not for me.

19. Life will be different and you can handle that. In fact, many things improve.

20. Don't get sucked in to believing there's a "new normal." Nothing about the process feels normal. I hate that phrase.

21. If you don't want to call yourself a survivor, don't. Don't let labels define your recovery.

22. Write a book or tell your story to help those experiencing cancer for the first time or are having a recurrence.

23. Be kind to yourself every chance you get.

24. Don't expect others to understand your struggle. You barely understand yourself.

25. Don't expect doctors to have all the answers. Be hungry for information and steadfast about getting quality information.

26. Speak up whenever possible for fundraising efforts for cancers of all types, especially the rare ones because they have the least amount of funding. Please include fundraisers for companion animals too.

27. Lend your efforts to groups that focus on helping those less fortunate than yourself.

28. Be thankful The Affordable Care Act was enacted so you will be allowed to get insurance coverage and not be disqualified or denied coverage. You were born at a good time.

29. Do your ancestry.com work and find out what genetic predispositions you might have for cancers of all kinds. Don't let negative history repeat itself if at all possible.

30. Eat great food.

31. Spend quality time with friends and family.

32. Laugh out loud and laugh often.

33. Appreciate every moment you're not barfing...oh, did I already say that?

34. Before and/or after chemotherapy make every effort to find out what toxins you are carrying around inside your body and work on getting them out as soon as possible.

35. When in doubt, hug people.

36. Know a little about everyone's jobs because you will need to know if they are doing it correctly.

37. It may be hard to trust people during the journey. Develop a key sense of discernment that doesn't shut *everyone* out. Someone might have great ideas for you.

38. Learn how to forget things.

39. Get the help you need to desensitize yourself to the trauma you have endured.

40. Celebrate each and every encouraging result.

41. Never lose sight of the importance of really kind and generous people. They are the angels amongst us.

42. Be open with your story for it may help someone who is suffering in silence.

43. There will be a time when you will feel like your story has been told enough times and you can retire it. It will be a sure sign you are healing.

44. Keep dreaming of better days ahead.

45. Know that sometimes you just have to do stuff you don't want to do.

46. Sometimes it's best to just close your eyes and not look at some things.

47. Smile when your heart is aching. Smile when you feel like breaking. Just smile.

48. Keep your pets close by. They seem to understand, and they enjoy hanging out, A LOT.

49. Don't expect the insurance company to understand your struggle.

50. When nauseous, limit the viewing of food related TV shows.

51. Remember that as long as you're alive you ARE alive.

52. Enjoy the fact that you may lose some not-so-shiny friends during the process.

53. Realize that your physical body and image will change during your journey, but don't let that ruin a perfectly good opportunity to feel beautiful as often as possible.

54. Always, always know that you can contact me by going to www.annekrusethewriter.com or by e-mailing me directly at annekrusewriter@gmail.com if you have any questions, concerns or great jokes. If you've had cancer, I would love to hear about the top three things you learned through the cancer journey. I hope to gather a compilation of wisdoms and share them with the world.

55. Always bring dessert, unless someone is nauseous.

56. Don't read the obituaries during treatment; or simply stop all together.

57. Identify "measures of recovery" so you will know that you are making progress. For example, when you are able to put away a particular medication because you don't need it anymore.

58. The insurance company may not pay for the very thing that you've needed to stop the relentless nausea you might be experiencing.

59. Medicinal marijuana may disappoint you.

60. You will eventually return to receiving less than great customer service at your doctor's office, which is a sign that things are improving.

61. Don't fight every battle that comes your way. Choose wisely based on energy expenditures and realistic outcomes.

62. If you have benefitted from an unconventional form of treatment be prepared for others including doctors, dentists, nurses, friends and family to look at you funny.

63. You will hear people tell you, "At least you're alive," as a way to quiet you when you bring a problematic side effect to their attention. Note: Just say, "I know, hallelujah!" and

then continue to tell them about the side effect because they may learn something from you that may help another patient.

64. Don't wait for your M.D. to talk about or treat you for things related to your rejuvenation after they complete their portion of your treatment. You must seek and find a group of talented healthcare professionals to help you. They're out there.

65. When you read discouraging news or hear a discouraging story just put your blinders on and focus on your individual efforts to get healthy.

66. Limit your Google research time to twenty minutes on any one ailment.

67. Your condition and prognosis may change as time goes on. Mentally prepare ahead of time by remembering that your situation can be like renovating a house: it's always 20 percent more "expensive" than expected and it will likely take longer than anticipated.

68. If you go home with a catheter make sure they know what side of the bed you sleep on so the bag can be adhered to the correct side of your hip.

69. Going through terrifying Halloween mazes will help prepare you for entering the infusion center for chemotherapy.

70. Thank your radiation technicians and infusion center workers every day you see them because it will help mark the completion of each treatment and help you focus on getting through the course.

71. The fun part about the cancer journey is getting to be really choosy about with whom you spend time. You've had cancer, and you may find yourself shuffling, categorizing and prioritizing your relationships in a way that allows you to only spend quality time with quality people for quality reasons.

72. Others may not know what to do for you, with you or know how to behave around you, and that's okay. Just breathe.

73. Get your hands on a good banana bread recipe. It's a great comfort food and great to quell nausea.

74. The feeling of relief will become one of your favorite feelings because it's the opposite of dread.

75. Make follow-up appointments one month ahead to allow time to mentally prepare for the appointment. Establish a routine for relaxation and positive self-talk leading up to your appointment, and in the doctor's office lobby and waiting room.

76.   The art of disconnecting from your feelings is also important to have in your hip pocket when you need it. Don't use it too often.

77.   Make sure you ask the doctor if they took a sewing class in junior high because the lack of that skill will ensure a hideous scar like mine.

78.   My best advice during the period of recovery and rejuvenation is to be informed,   keep good records and put those records away where you won't have to see them or think about them until it's time to make the next follow-up appointment.

79.   You are your own case study. Enjoy the education.

80.   Read as much as you can.

81.   Scrutinize articles from respected journals, university-based books, and internet information with a keen eye for checking sources and valid measures of correctness.

82.   Take responsibility for keeping your doctors informed of things that you know will impact your treatment.

83.   Cancer allows you to reset the clock on just about every aspect of your life. Make wise choices about those changes.

84.   You may find yourself struggling to find a way to shift from feeling disgusted about your body to feeling worthy of being desired. The simple wisdom is to be kind to yourself and purposefully participate in those things that allow a cathartic and transformative experience.

85.   The investment of time and money you put into your own rejuvenation will be the best money you have ever spent. You're worth it – period.

86.   You will have medical bills to pay even though your insurance company covers your treatment. That's why people write books to make money to pay them off.

87.   Writing a book to pay those bills is the equivalent to giving cancer the finger because you found a way to make money to kill a monster.

88.   You may need to help others be comfortable around you.

89.   Don't stay too long in your private little cave; mildew will set in.

90.   You can empty a room sometimes just by mentioning death and cancer, which isn't always a bad thing.

91.   Try to put the idea of attending a follow-up appointment out of your head, but always set your phone alarm to remind you 24 hours ahead of your appointment. Don't miss appointments.

92. Tell unsmiling staff at doctor's office, "Don't smile or your face will crack." They usually smile. If not, walk away smiling.

93. Be present and accountable at all your appointments.

94. Vaccines for cervical cancer only protect against cervical cancer caused by HPV. These account for only 85 percent of cases, which means 15 percent are non-HPV related. Don't fool yourself into a false sense of security just because you or your daughters are vaccinated. Don't forget your sons because they can get HPV too and later in life pass it along to women.

95. If you have a special dog, he or she could earn a Therapy Dog Certification and visit people in the chemo infusion center. Animals bring comfort to a lot of people.

96. Watch out for nurses named, Agnes.

97. When life gives you a scar, make art out of it.

98. When in doubt, see a doctor about it.

99. Don't poo-poo yourself into thinking every health ailment is due to hormones.

100. Don't always believe your thoughts are true especially when you're under a lot of pressure and under the influence of a controlled substance.

101. You will show yourself you are braver than you ever thought you were. Anything you do in the future will seem totally doable in comparison.

"Live Life To Write About It." – Anne Kruse

THE LAST PAGE

I was always that person who flipped to the last page of a book to see how things turned out. Juvenile wisdom convinced me that somehow I would be able to understand the ending without experiencing the entire book. Usually a book report deadline was looming, and the threat of a horrible grade to mar my academic record. I don't do that anymore because I enjoy watching a story build and characters reveal themselves through the twists and turns as the black ink lays claim on the white page.

Right now I'm hoping that you have read the Introduction, it hooked you like a meat cleaver, you read the entire book and you are merely reading this page because we are coming to the end of our journey together. I'm so grateful for the opportunity to tell my story and for you to read it.

If you are reading this page before reading the book, may the mere thought of doing so intrigue you and capture your every thought to the point of compelling you to turn back to the Introduction and start your journey. If that syrupy passage didn't spark your sweet tooth, then thank you for visiting my book. Have a wonderful day. Hope to see you soon.

The act of writing this book has been fulfilling in so many ways; most importantly it helped me write my way out of a slump and find my writing voice again. Cancer surgery pilfered the organs associated with creative energy, so I wondered how it would affect my ability to write. It feels incredible to be making some noise and to be heard again.

My college basketball coach, the late, great Colleen Riley, taught me the only way out of a shooting slump is to shoot. It takes courage and a lot of shooting. It took a lot of courage and writing to revive what I thought cancer had silenced. Coach Riley passed away in August of 2011 from pancreatic cancer, and I was diagnosed with cervical cancer just four months later. Seeing her journey was both inspiring and incredibly sad. She was an icon to me and to many, many others. Witnessing others go into battle before you can help you tap into courage you didn't even know you had. She set the stage for so many people throughout her life, and even in her death she continues to inspire. If this book does for others just a smidgen of what she did for me, then I could not be happier.

I decided to price the book to make it as accessible as possible to anyone who needs or wants the information. Although it will be in tiny little increments, the proceeds will go toward cancer research. Let me clarify: I've spent a lot of money *researching* ways to improve my health during my entire journey, which has been a bit costly. Thus, earnings from this book will help pay off the huge financial debt cancer left in my lap. Paying off the balance will symbolize an enormous victory over cancer. I thank you in advance for contributing to my success. My hope is that you appreciate my efforts to write a book to fight "the monster" rather than simply ask for a hand-out. However, feel free to donate if you are so inclined at www.annekrusethewriter.com

I've used my story, writing skills, my mental, emotional and physical resources to create this book to serve others, and it feels incredible.

One of my lofty goals is to get this book added to the REQUIRED textbook list for every medical school, nursing school, counseling program, medical assistant program, and writer's program and film school. It would be a great addition to the library of every cancer recovery group, and to the waiting room of every oncologist's offices. While I'm at it, why not make it an impulse buy at every pharmacy counter and every coffee fueling station? I want it to be in the hands of those who want to know what it's like and what to expect, and to see that I made it through, and so can they.

PLEASE E-MAIL ME SHOULD YOU HAVE A LEAD TO CONTACT TO HELP ME ACHIEVE MY LOFTY GOAL: annekrusewriter@gmail.com

I realize some of the subject matter in this book shines a light on less-than-positive employee behaviors within the medical community. It was my intent to discuss these incidents to illuminate "teaching opportunities" that are alive and well and must be addressed. All of us are faced with challenges in our work environment. Those who interact with delightfully diverse populations, in varied and complex situations, galvanize the need for constant learning.

This experience has deepened my capacity to understand the human condition, which allows for more interesting and fully developed fictional characters in my future writing projects. A writer's journey through cancer is unique because a writer can express the things so many people can't put into words, but wish they could. Creating an extremely relatable experience for an audience is every writer's ultimate ambition.

I would like to include a special note to writers. My focus on the structural storytelling components of my trek ensured the presence of: an inciting incident, reversals, a point-of-no-return, internal dilemmas becoming externalized, the "whiff of death" moment, a legitimate third act, and a satisfying ending. There is a likable protagonist, me, who experiences a punishing emotional arc. As for a life-threatening antagonist, cancer is one of the few guaranteed shoe-ins.

Conventional wisdom recommends that writers write what they know. What if you are asked, and hopefully paid, to develop a character that has experienced cancer when you have not? That's why writers need to buy this book. It will expand your resume's potential – period; and will support a fellow writer. Go team!

I am proud to say I have finished this book and now the story will live on forever. For that, I do kind of feel like a superhero. Cancer Girl writes her book and saves the world, with an ample amount of special effects and a kickass crew by her side, of course.

As far as what I will be doing next: I'll be writing anything and everything I can; but the best way to put it is to say,

"To be continued …"

I'll be busy living the dot, dot, dot, and writing all about it.

On that note, I WOULD LOVE FOR YOU TO WRITE A REVIEW OF MY BOOK on the Amazon website. It will help my cause and probably make you feel pretty good too.

Once you are in go to BOOKS > Type in ANNE KRUSE > CLICK on the title of my book > on the product page CLICK on WRITE A REVIEW just under the title. It will only take a minute. Thank you in advance for a SPECTACULAR REVIEW (hint-hint).

While you're at it please take a pic of yourself reading my book and share it on Facebook, **Instagram**, pin it on Pinterest, connect with me on **LinkedIn**, and even tie a note to a pigeon's foot and send it to a friend to help me get the word out. I've got world-wide goals!

Please visit www.annekrusethewriter.com should you need writing services, career counseling services and to stay abreast of my projects.

My children's book, *Takota's Dream* is available on my site as well.

"Live Life To Write About It." – Anne Kruse

ON THE COVER

I experimented with a practical, yet artistic approach to create a mental shift in my thinking that I hoped would encourage healing. It ended up as the cover art for this book. Turning a part of me I viewed as "EW" into something NEW and artfully expressive, was pure transformation. A crooked and gathered eleven-inch scar jags its way down the majority of my abdomen. I took a photograph of my scar (a "scarfy" – a selfie of my scar) and uploaded it into Photoshop. I sectioned off portions of my scar and surrounding shadow variations then playfully painted each without too much deep thought. The canvas was quickly filled. You might notice a little bit of the scar peeking through the design. This was intentional and represents the notion that **reality doesn't go away; but we can change our perception.** What resulted from my experiment was art, or what I call, SCART. It was art therapy at its best. It left me feeling like it wasn't a scar, but rather a beautiful, well-earned badge of honor.

www.ingramcontent.com/pod-product-compliance
Lightning Source LLC
Chambersburg PA
CBHW051909170526
45168CB00001B/302